PILATES-BASED EXERCISES FOR LIFETIME FITNESS

Judy Bloomquist
Texas A&M University, Kingsville

Darlene Stockton
Coastal Bend College

american press
60 STATE STREET #700
BOSTON, MASSACHUSETTS 02109

CONTENTS

PREFACE

Exercise has come a long way in the 21st century. There are new innovative forms of exercise being discovered and invented to make the whole exercise process as simple as possible for people of all ages and fitness levels while attempting to reduce the risk for injury and impact to the body. Pilates is one of those forms of exercise. We as college instructors recognized the usefulness and positive aspects of incorporating this form of exercise into our college activity class offerings. However, when attempting to find a college textbook that teaches Pilates and its history to our students we were unable to find a match. We do not claim to be experts in this field but do have many hours of experience performing and teaching the exercises and have become very excited to pass on the knowledge and benefits to be gained from participating in Pilates to others.

Both of us hold Masters Degrees in Kinesiology. We began working together in 2005 which inspired the creation of this book. Currently Darlene Stockton is teaching at Coastal Bend College in Beeville, Texas and Judy Bloomquist is teaching at Texas A&M University-Kingsville, Texas. Our goal is to provide our students with the information and instruction necessary for them to understand the importance of being fit and staying fit throughout life, long after their college experience is over.

We would like to extend our special thanks to Della De La Garza for all her hard work and assistance in completing this project and D.J. Poland for posing for pictures.

Judy Bloomquist
Darlene Stockton

Chapter One

INTRODUCTION TO PILATES

There are many forms and techniques of exercise introduced regularly with many programs fading out as fast as they were born. Pilates has stood the test of time. Fitness is no longer a means of survival in society today. Our world has become so high-tech and so fast-paced that our survival skills now include being able to point and click a computer mouse or send a text message rather than hunting and gathering food as in the past. That is why it is imperative that we each find some form of exercise that fits into our busy lifestyles.

Pilates (puh-la-tees) is becoming more and more popular. Pilates is a form of exercise that helps to strengthen and tone muscles, increase coordination, build muscular endurance, and improve flexibility and posture with less chance of injury which can occur from resistance training and weight bearing exercises. This is accomplished by using controlled flowing movements as the mind and body work together. Many people make the mistake of trying to get fit within a matter of weeks after being inactive for years. Setting unrealistic goals and trying to progress at too fast of a pace is a set up for failure and can even result in injuries. Exercise should be beneficial; therefore, it is important to approach any exercise program with the appropriate knowledge that will prevent the mistakes that could hinder progress in reaching desired outcomes and goals.

There are four reasons why a person may want to consider a Mat Pilates exercise program. First, a mat Pilates class is very time efficient and can produce a full body workout in a short period of time. Many people have the mentality "if a little is good; more is better." In the past quantity instead of quality exercise was stressed too often. Today with lack of time being given as the major reason for not exercising, it makes perfect sense to stress a quality exercise program that can be performed in less time while providing a workout that will produce results. The average Pilates class is 45 minutes to 1 hour, but we believe that 30 minutes of well planned exercises can be equally beneficial because many of these exercises target multiple muscle groups with each maneuver. Most people have heard the term "multi-tasking," this is what Pilates accomplishes even though the main focus is on the core muscles.

The second reason for considering Mat-Based Pilates is that according to Joseph H. Pilates and W.J. Miller, everyone can perform and benefit from the participation of Pilates exercises (Your Health, p.11). In addition, Pilates may help prevent injuries by maintaining a strong healthy body. In the early 20th century dancers embraced Joseph Pilates' exercise program after realizing that it was possible for a dancer to continue exercising during the healing process without risking further damage to the existing injury. Dancers considered the fluid movements to be aesthetic (Menezes, 2000). Dancers found they could maintain their conditioning while rehabilitating the injury. This allowed the dancer to reach that "peak" performance condition in a shorter period of time after resuming their normal dance sessions. Therefore, it is possible for average people with injuries to benefit from Pilates exercises during the rehabilitation process without impact on the joints. It is always best to consult your physician before beginning a new exercise program especially if there are pre-existing injuries.

The third reason for choosing Pilates is that the exercises can be designed to meet the needs of all fitness levels. This allows the individual to work at their own fitness level and progress at their own pace. For example, while performing a seated forward toe touch, one person may reach to the toes and another may only reach to the knees to accomplish the purpose of the exercise. Another example would be while performing the "one hundred," one person may be positioned with a 90-degree angle at the hip and another may be working more intensely with a greater angle at the hip. The "no pain—no gain" mentality is taken out of the equation. Discomfort may be experienced due to the contracting of the muscles resulting in muscle fatigue; however, physical pain is virtually eliminated. Anytime a person experiences a sharp pain it is a signal that something may be wrong and the exercise should be re-evaluate to make sure that the technique and alignment are correct to insure the desired outcome and to prevent injuries. Control of all bodily movements is stressed. This enhances the individual's kinesthetic awareness of the body and what it is capable of doing. This awareness further serves to decrease the chance of injury.

Finally, the fourth reason for considering Pilates-based exercises is that it can be done by all ages. Once this method of exercising has been learned, it can easily be performed at home or while traveling due to the minimal equipment, time, and space requirements. The Pilates-based mat exercise workout can be modified to accommodate virtually any schedule and setting allowing continual benefits for all who use the program. If you maintain a strong, healthy body and mind you not only increase the chance for a longer life, you also enhance the quality of life.

Pilates based mat exercises condition the mind and the body. The mind and body must work together as our mind controls our muscles. After teaching our classes each semester there are several reoccurring comments made by the students:

1. "I find myself sitting up straighter in my classes."
2. "I feel a difference already."
3. "I did not realize I would get this much of a workout."
4. "My clothes fit me better now."

When you look in on a Pilates-based mat class, it can be a little deceiving. The participants are usually lying on the floor, and are not out of breath or sweating profusely. However, when this workout is properly executed, it can be very intense. Pilates-based mat classes can be done simply with a yoga mat or with additional equipment such as an exercise ball, hand weights, bars, resistance bands and tubing, and rings, for added resistance and variety. The popularity of Mat Pilates classes and the interest in this form of exercise continues to grow in the college setting and in the fitness club setting which is well reflected in the availability of videos and teaching materials on the market today.

Chapter Two
THE CREATOR

The name Pilates comes from its creator, Joseph Hubertus Pilates (1880–1967). Joseph Pilates was born in Germany and as a young boy suffered from a variety of health problems such as rickets, asthma, and rheumatic fever. Even though he became very weak from these conditions he was determined to strengthen and condition his body. By the age of fourteen he was studying the musculoskeletal system of the human body in addition to the movement of the human and animal bodies. During his teenage years he overcame his frailties and successfully conditioned his body, as a result he was asked to pose for professional anatomical drawings and was considered a prime specimen (Menezes, 2000). Joseph Pilates studied Eastern forms of exercise that included yoga, Zen, meditation and the early governmental systems of the ancient Greek and Roman militaries while developing his own method of training and exercise. He combined the techniques of the Eastern and Western exercise to emerge with today's method known as "Pilates."

In 1912 Joseph Pilates toured England as a boxer and a circus performer. There seems to be some confusion as to the reason that he was touring England. During his time in England, World War I broke out and he was detained along with other German Nationals. It was while he was working in one of Britain's military camps that he started to develop a form of mat work that became known as "contrology" which eventually took on the name of Pilates. He was in a second military camp; this is where he became a caregiver of bedridden patients and began to develop specialized equipment to aid in their rehabilitation.

After the war, Joseph Pilates went back to Germany where he began a career as a personal trainer for the military police teaching self-defense. Joseph Pilates was not happy with the politics of Germany and decided to migrate to the United States in 1926. He met his wife to be, Clara, on the ship in route. She suffered from arthritis so he used his methods to help her regain her strength. He brought his method of exercise to the states with hopes of influencing the dancing world. Joseph and Clara opened a dance studio in New York City. His ideas were both welcomed and embraced by the New York City Ballet Company where he continued to develop his "contrology" until his death in 1967. His wife Clara continued using and teaching his method of mat exercises. He is considered a man who devoted his life to fitness.

Chapter Three

GENERAL FITNESS

Pilates exercise programs are becoming more and more popular and most individuals can participate in this type of program. However, it is important that the participant be familiar with general fitness factors so they can avoid mistakes to prevent discouragement. There is no magic type of exercise that will address all the components of fitness. This can only be accomplished by a variety of activities. Our bodies were designed to be physically active not sedentary. It is when we quit using our bodies that the problems begin.

Many people start an exercise program because they want to lose weight. Typically, the adherence rate to these programs is not good. Many people do not arm themselves with the knowledge necessary to succeed and often fail in reaching their goals. Weight loss goals must be realistic and based on scientific principles. Most people believe in calorie input versus output. This is true, but any weight loss program that does not include exercise could result in the loss of lean mass. This is a critical issue that needs to be addressed. There are many advertisements that promise weight loss and even rapid weight loss. Some of these ads seem to suggest that the pounds almost melt away by just taking a pill. If that were possible there would not be overweight people or an obesity epidemic. Approximately two pounds per week is considered a realistic safe weight loss (Kravitz, 2006). This is best accomplished by a balanced diet and regular exercise. Drinking more water, reducing sugar consumption, reducing intake of saturated fat, and eating food products that are not highly processed is a good beginning.

Before you start your exercise program it is important to have a physical or consult a doctor if prior health conditions exist. The purpose of exercise is to make you feel better; therefore, it is imperative that any underlying problems, concerns and/or health and safety risks should be addressed before beginning an exercise program.

Often the hardest phase of an exercise program is getting started and making up your mind to actually begin. Once you have that initial first day under your belt it is a little easier to continue especially for those that have not exercised in a long time. Exercise should not be painful, but it may involve some discomfort. Many times people who experience physical discomfort that is associated with exercise report that they feel better mentally and physically after a bout of exercise. It is important to remember that we do not get out of shape in one day; therefore, we can not get back into shape in one day either. It is beneficial to start slow, and then increase the amount of exercise being done. Once the body has adapted to lower intensity levels of the exercises the overload principle can be applied which increases the intensity levels by performing more advanced poses.

The "buddy system" is strongly recommended. Having a workout companion often motivates individuals to continue exercising on a regular basis. This concept is especially beneficial when a plateau occurs and may make a difference between quitting and continuing the exercise program.

There are a few general fitness factors that are important that participants should know in order to participate in any exercise program safely and to promote the attainment of set goals. There are five components of fitness. All five of these components should be addressed in a fitness program to achieve total fitness. It is important to choose specific activities that are enjoyable and meet the criteria of each component. Total fitness requires addressing all of the components which will equal a well rounded program that includes variety.

Aerobic and **anaerobic** are two terms that you should consider prior to beginning your Mat Pilates based exercise program. Aerobic means with oxygen and should be rhythmic, involve the large muscles groups be at least 20 minutes or longer and be vigorous enough to elevate the heart rate. Examples would be *power walking, running/jogging, swimming, aerobic dance classes, or cycling/spinning (spinning is class format). Anaerobic exercise means without oxygen and involves the bodily systems that do not require the presence of oxygen to produce energy. Examples include Pilates-based exercises, yoga, weight training, calisthenics, and sprinting. It is recognized that these systems are not always one or the other; it is possible to combine the two. Some activities such as basketball, racquetball, or squash require these energy producing systems to work together (Kravitz, 2006).

THE FIVE COMPONENTS OF FITNESS

1. **Cardiorespiratory fitness** is the ability of the heart, lungs, and blood vessels to supply oxygen to the working muscles to sustain movement for a period of time.

A key part of this definition is "sustain movement for a period of time." There are two questions that need to be addressed:

Question #1 is "What type of activity?"
Question #2 is "How long should I stay active?"

Any activity that utilizes **aerobic exercise** is appropriate. Aerobic exercise promotes fat loss. Pilates-based exercises do not incorporate this component of fitness, but still offer many health benefits. Success with exercise programs depends on choosing activities that involve rhythmic movement of the larger muscle groups and are enjoyable. Beginners may not be able to continue an activity for 20 minutes when first starting out. It is important to not get discouraged as it is okay to start slowly and gradually increase the length of time of the activity. It is also very important not to over exercise especially in the beginning because it may lead to early burnout. General recommendations for aerobic exercise are 30 minutes three times per week for cardiovascular benefits and four to five days per week for weight loss (Kravitz, 2006). The exercise program should progress up to the desired time and number of days according to each individual's fitness level. Doing this and letting the body adapt may aid in the continuance of the program. The exercise program will build up to the desired time and the desired number of days with progression.

One type of cardiovascular activity includes Power Walking. It is a style of walking that involves the use of the upper body (much like in running) as well as the legs. The goal is to move forward avoiding any crossing over of the arms (neither arm should cross the mid line of the body). The feet strike the ground in front of each foot (picture an imaginary line between the feet, each foot strikes on its respective side) unlike race walking (the imaginary line between the feet and each foot would strike the line). Some people have a hard time walking fast making it hard to elevate the heart rate so you may want to concentrate on the arms moving faster rather than the legs moving faster. When you do this the legs will follow, speeding up the pace.

2. **Muscular Strength** is the ability of a muscle or muscle group to exert maximum force in a single effort.

   As we age and become less active we begin to lose muscle mass (atrophy). This factor can affect the quality of life in our senior years. Each one of us should make a conscious effort to maintain strong muscles. A small amount of strength training (This does not mean starting a body building program) will yield long term health benefits. However, many women tend to avoid strength training due to a fear of developing extensive muscle mass and enlargement (hypertrophy). Technology encourages society to be less active with the increased use of computers, TV, riding lawn mowers, hands free vacuum cleaners; therefore, it becomes an individual responsibility to prevent the loss of lean mass. Pilates addresses muscular strength with the use of our body weight as resistance and using multiple muscle groups to maintain balance and posture throughout the exercise. The muscles are strengthened but not in the same way heavy resistance training does. An important fact is that the more lean mass you have the more calories your body will burn when exercising and when at rest (Kravitz, 2006). Muscle mass increases the body's metabolic rate.

3. **Muscular Endurance** is the ability of the muscle or muscle group to contract repeatedly or to hold a contraction of submaximal force over a period of time.

It has been documented that if you strength train there will be an increase in muscular strength as well as muscular endurance to some extent, but there is little increase seen in strength gains when working on muscular endurance (Hale, 2005). Pilates increases muscular endurance and is based on the number of repetitions or length of time contractions are held.

4. **Flexibility** is the range of motion of a joint.

Flexibility is joint specific which means that the flexibility at each joint varies. For example a person may be very flexible in the right shoulder, but not in the left. There are many factors that affect flexibility; for example, injury to the joint, tearing of muscles tissue, injured connective tissue, and obesity. Maintaining flexibility is essential to your quality of life. Flexibility may lessen the chance of injury but should not be taken to extreme by over-stretching which results in loss of joint stability. There are several forms of stretching. This book addresses only two: Static and Ballistic stretching. Static stretching is considered safe method compared to ballistic stretching that has been linked to injuries. Ballistic stretching uses bouncing and/or jerky movements to increase muscle length. This increases the chance of a muscle strain and tears. Static stretching involves slowly moving into a position and holding that position for a period of time. There may be some discomfort when stretching, but stretching should never involve sharp pain. If the muscle group begins to shake while stretching the intensity of the stretch should be reduced slightly to avoid injury (Wuest & Bucher, 2006).

A common mistake often made is that some use stretching exercises as a form of warm-up. The term warm-up implies increasing the body's core temperature to allow the muscles to become warm and supple which enables them to lengthen slowly and naturally (Mayoclinic.com, 2005).

There is some controversy regarding the perfect time to stretch; after the warm-up, after the workout is completed, or both. The best advice is to listen to your body and to err on the safe side by stretching after the warm-up and after the workout. If time does not allow for both it is best to stretch after the workout (Mayoclinic.com, 2995). Stretching after the warm-up normally involves less time and will not be as intense as the stretches after the workout. It is thought that most flexibility gains are made after the workout because the muscles are very warm and easier to stretch. Two other reasons for stretching at the end of the workout are for aiding in prevention of muscle soreness and to ensure a proper cool down.

5. **Body Composition** is the ratio of body fat to lean body mass. In the past we have used the scale and height/weight ratio charts to determine if we were over or under weight. The major problem with this formula is that it does not take into consideration the percentage of lean mass and body fat. In a comparison of two people weighing 150 pounds that are both 5'7" using the BMI index formula to determine if they fall with in healthy guidelines may give confusing results because both people would fall into the same category but may have body fat percentages that vary greatly. This drastically affects the health of a person with extreme body fat making him/her highly susceptible to heart disease and other hypokentic diseases.

The best way to achieve a good body composition is through exercise and a balanced diet. By severely reducing the caloric content of your diet you will retard your progress. Skipping meals or not eating three meals per day can also cause you metabolic rate to decline.

In order to prevent your body from storing the calories taken in instead of burning them, we must eat regularly. Many believe that five small meals per day rather than three larger meals per day may be more beneficial in regards to weight loss. When the body does not get fed for extended periods of time alarms go off within the body and it goes into a starvation mode. The body naturally begins to slow the metabolism and the rate at which calories are burned to attempt to ration and control energy levels. The body does not understand that you want it to use some of that stored energy (body fat) so that you can lose weight, but instead goes into a survival mode and stores a little extra for later. This is our body's way of preventing starvation. So those that try to eat only one or two meals per day are actually hindering their progress.

Your exercise program should include all the components of fitness and be based on the progressive overload principle. There are several ways to overload by increasing the frequency of the workouts, the intensity of the workouts, or the time length of the workouts. When increasing the overload choose only one of the three modifications (frequency, intensity and time).

FITT

FITT is an acronym for *Frequency, Intensity,* and *Time* and *Type*.

"F" stands for frequency and refers to how many days per week you exercise (3 days considered maintenance; 3 to 5 recommended). Pilates could be performed daily due to the low intensity and non-impact to the joints.

"I" stands for intensity and refers to how hard you exercise each time you exercise (cardiorespiratory uses target heart rates; perceived exertion method, and talk test to monitor intensity). Pilates offers many variations of intensity depending on the fitness level and health condition of the individual. This book demonstrates two or three different levels of intensity for most exercises and how to accomplish them.

"T" stands for time and refers to how long you exercise each time you exercise (may sometimes be referred to as duration). A full-body Pilates workout can be accomplished in 45 minutes to 1 hour if it is properly planned and organized.

The second *"T"* stands for type and is used to differentiate between aerobic and anaerobic types of exercise.

This Pilates-based workout is an anaerobic form of exercise. Although calories will be burned while the exercises are being performed, this workout is not a weight loss program. It is recommended that this workout be combined with some form of aerobic exercise to achieve the best overall fitness and health.

An example of the overload principle with a goal of weight loss consists of changing a 30-minute walk three times per week, to a 40-minute walk three times per week. Overload is accomplished by increasing the time.

Another example of applying overload consists of changing the intensity level by running an average of 3.0 miles in 20 minutes to begin with and progressing to 3.25 miles in 20 minutes. Overload is accomplished by increasing the speed.

It is important to never increase more than one of these variables at a time. This will help prevent early exhaustion and chronic injuries.

Circuit training and resistance ball exercises are two other formats that can be incorporated into any exercise program to offer a change of pace. (See Chapters 9 and 10).

Chapter Four

THE SIX PRINCIPLES OF PILATES

There are six basic principles that Joseph Pilates believed to be essential to his exercise program (Dillman, 2001). It is important that each of these principles be addressed to ensure safety and the desired results. Individuals that participate in a Pilates-based program will enhance body awareness.

1. **Concentration**
   - √ Mind and body connection
   - √ Mind initiates action
   - √ Listen to your body
   - √ Focus on feeling of working muscles

2. **Control**
   - √ Prevents injury
   - √ Promotes the desired results

3. **Centering**
   - √ Powerhouse (abdominals, lower back, hip and buttocks)
   - √ Powerhouse allows for stabilization
   - √ Energy comes from the powerhouse

4. **Fluidity**
   - √ Movements are flowing
   - √ No quick, jerky movements

5. **Precision**
   - √ Every movement has a purpose
   - √ Every instruction is important
   - √ Will become second nature with practice

6. **Breathing**
   - √ Oxygenates the blood
   - √ Eliminates stale air
   - √ Proper technique (in through the nose; out through the mouth)

Chapter Five

BREATHING AND WARM-UP

Breathing plays a major role in achieving results when performing Pilates exercises; therefore, it is crucial that it is done properly. Correct breathing oxygenates the blood and increases circulation (Ungaro, 2002). When done properly, it will become beneficial in everyday life situations for calming, focusing, and releasing tension in the body.

The proper form of breathing consists of inhaling through the nose slowly, cautiously and deeply while allowing your rib cage to expand upward. This is followed by a slow controlled exhale through the mouth releasing all the air from the lungs and diaphragm (Menezes, A. 2000). Breathing provides awareness of being calm, in control and triggers the release of tension and stress (Gavin, 2003). Continued steady, rhythmic breathing should be maintained through each and every exercise for best results. It is crucial to avoid holding the breath while performing Pilates-based exercises as it causes intrathoracic pressure to rise. This is called the Val Salva Maneuver and is very dangerous (Brown, Miller, Eason, 2006).

A proper warm-up prior to performing any exercise is necessary to prepare the muscles to be lengthened and strengthened without injury. The length and intensity of a warm-up should be proportional to the intensity of the workout being performed. Pilates is considered a low impact anaerobic form of exercise that should include a warm-up of approximately 3-7 minutes involving the core muscles, shoulders, arms, and legs (Kravitz, 2006).

In addition to demonstrated warm-up exercises we have included the following list of alternative warm-up exercises not pictured that may help prepare the body for performing mat-based Pilates:

- shoulder shrugs
- shoulder rolls forward and backward

- head rolls or circles
- arm circles forward and backward
- toe taps
- heel raises
- walking/jogging

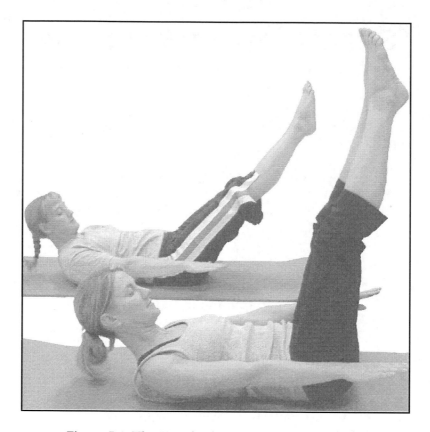

Figure 5.1: The Hundred and Advanced Hundred

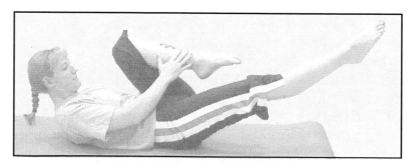

Figure 5.2: Single Leg Pump

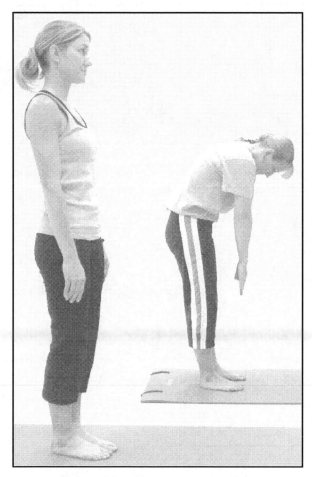

Figure 5.3: Standing Spinal Rolls

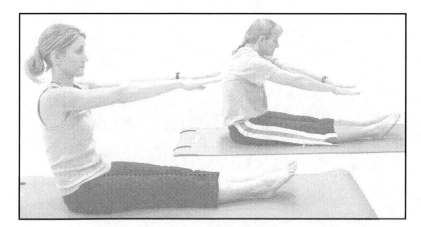

Figure 5.4: Seated Spinal Rolls

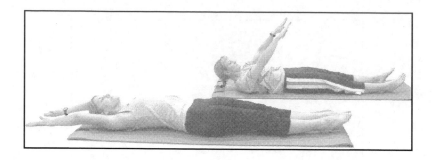

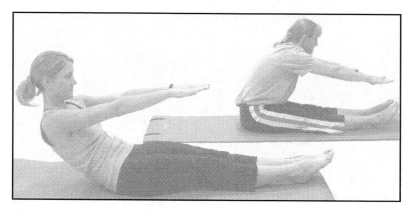

Figure 5.5a & b: The Roll Up

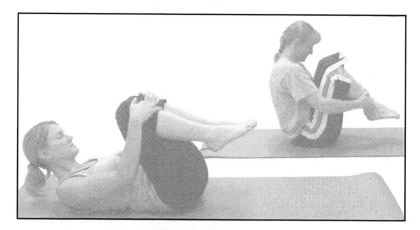

Figure 5.6: Roll Like a Ball

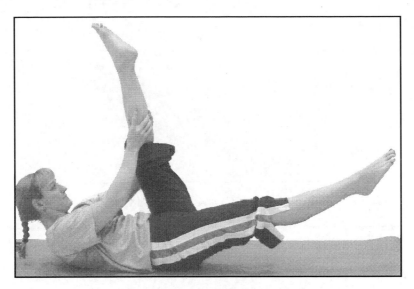

Figure 5.7: Scissors

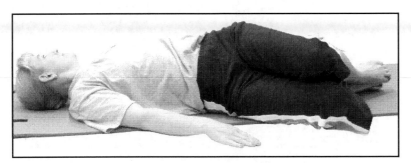

Figure 5.8: Torso Twist

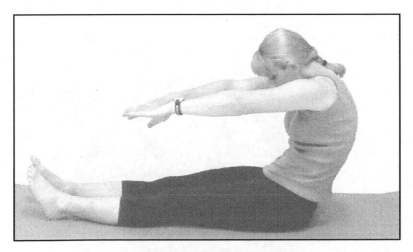

Figure 5.9: Seated "C" Curve

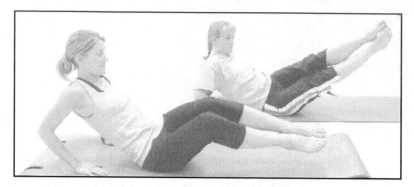

Figure 5.10: Can-Can & Extended Can-Can

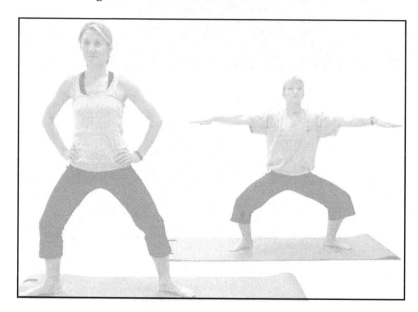

Figure 5.11: Plié

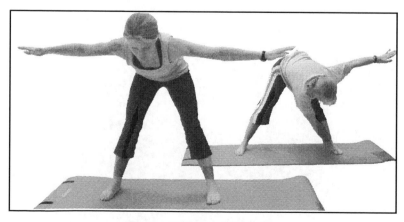

Figure 5.12: Arm Sweeps

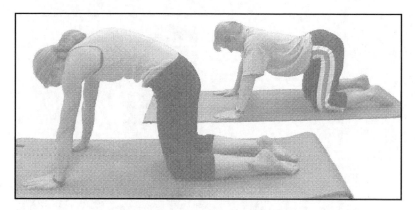

Figure 5.13: Cat Back Stretch

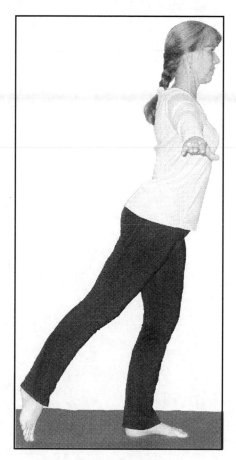

**Figure 5.14: Leg Sweeps
Forward and Back**

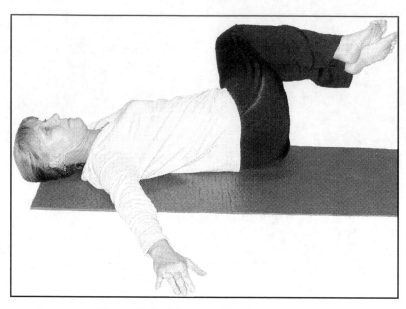

Figure 5.15: Knee Rolls Side to Side

Chapter Six

CORE EXERCISES

The following are exercises that target the "core" muscles which consist of the combination of abdominal and back muscles. These exercises are considered toning and require muscular endurance; therefore, the number of repetitions should not exceed the individual's personal fitness level. Mat-based Pilates exercising does not follow the concept of "No pain-No gain." The exercises should be performed without feeling pain or causing injury. These exercises are progressive starting at the beginning level and building up to the advanced moves. Each of these exercises should be executed with slow and controlled motion to avoid momentum assisting your muscles. In addition, it is crucial to maintain deep, slow, rhythmic breathing while performing exercises to ensure a calm and controlled workout. Proper form and technique are more important than the number of repetitions performed.

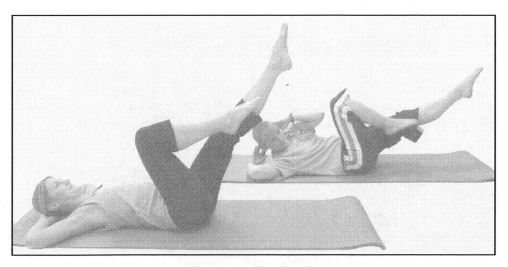

Figure 6.1: The Bicycle

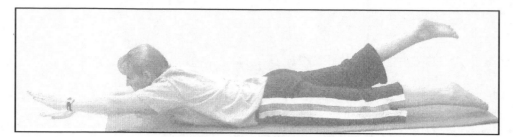

Figure 6.2: The Swimmer

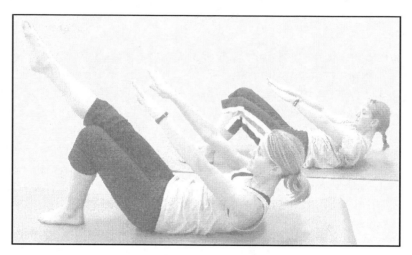

Figure 6.3: Bent Leg Roll Up and Advanced Version

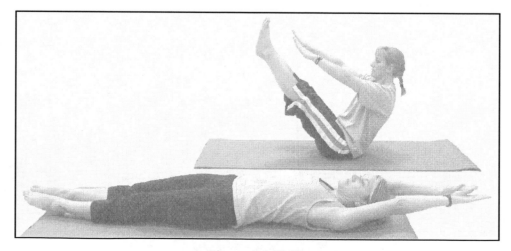

Figure 6.4: V Sit

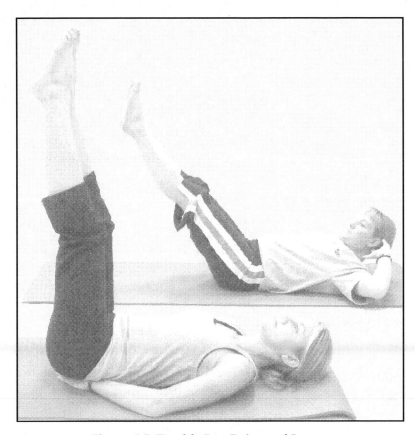

Figure 6.5: Double Leg Raise and Lower

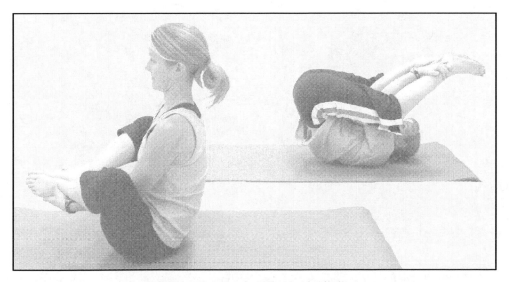

Figure 6.6: Seal with Heel Clicks

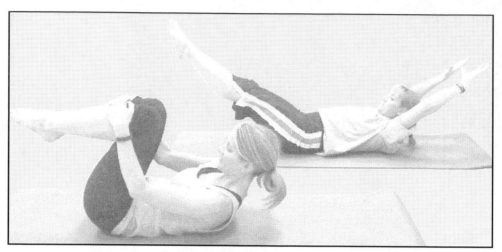

Figure 6.7: Blooming Flower

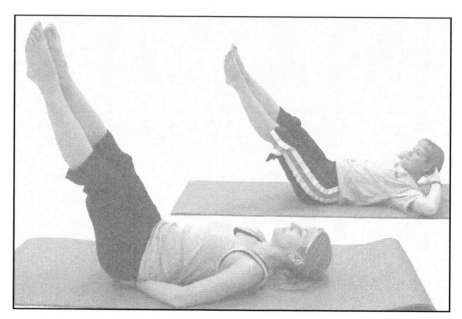

Figure 6.8: Corkscrew

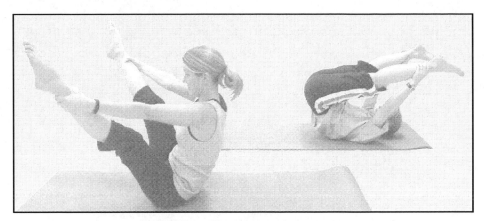

Figure 6.9: Open Leg Rocker

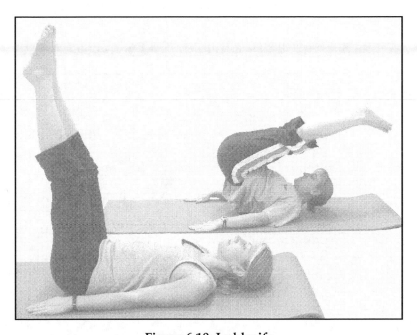

Figure 6.10: Jackknife

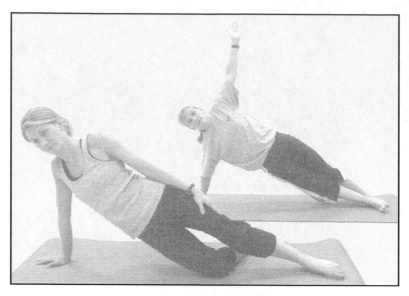

Figure 6.11: Side Plank

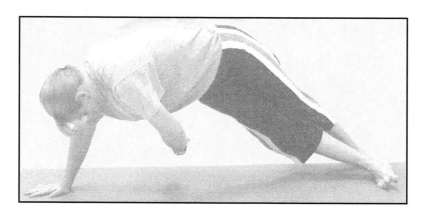

Figure 6.12: Advanced Side Plank with Scoop

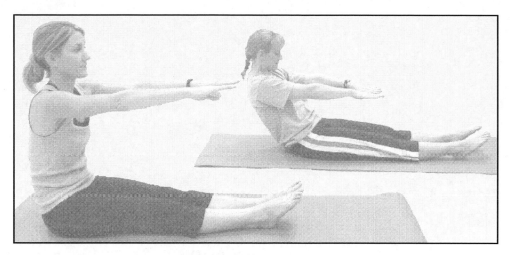

Figure 6.13: Phase I Rowing

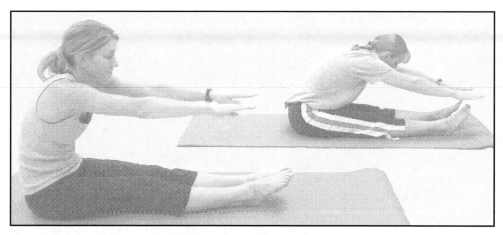

Figure 6.14: Phase II Rowing

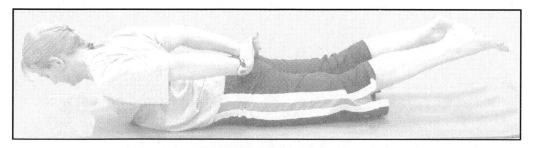

Figure 6.15: Mermaid

Chapter Seven

UPPER AND LOWER BODY EXERCISES

The following are exercises that target the upper and lower body muscle groups. These exercises are also considered toning and endurance in nature just as the exercises in Chapter Six; therefore, the number of repetitions should be consistent with the number of repetitions performed for core exercises. This number should also not exceed the person's individual fitness level. These exercises are also progressive and show beginner levels in addition to advanced levels for future challenges. It is important to remember that the breathing technique remains the same when performing any mat-based Pilates exercises.

The core muscle groups are also working during the upper and lower body exercises attempting to keep the body stable and preventing rolling around on the mat. Slow and controlled motions allow the muscles to do 100% of the work instead of flinging the arms and legs about which allows momentum to assist in doing the work or the motion being carried out.

Some of the upper and lower body exercises are pictured with additional equipment such as hand weights and/or an exercise ball for extra resistance and challenges; however, the following exercises may be performed just as effectively without the additional equipment until fitness levels improve.

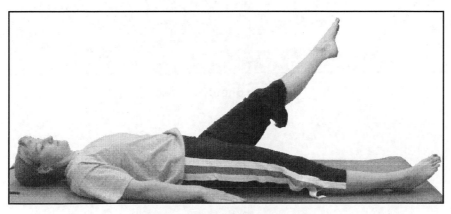

Figure 7.1: Single Leg Circles

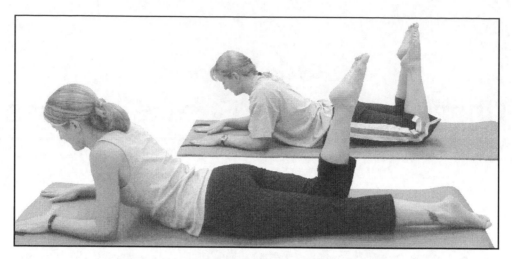

Figure 7.2: Single and Double Leg Kickbacks

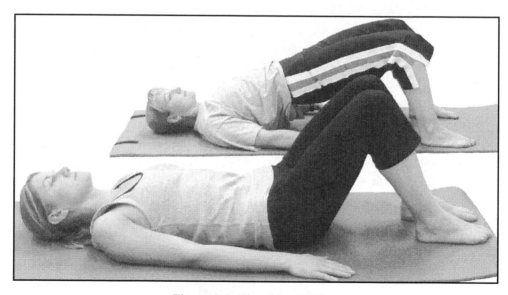

Figure 7.3: Shoulder Bridge

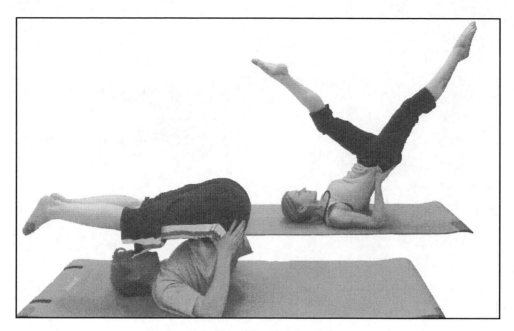

Figure 7.4: Shoulder Bridge Scissors

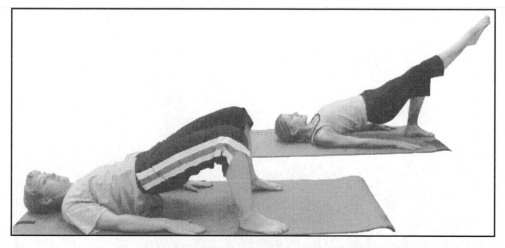

Figure 7.5: Beginning Should Bridge and Advanced Shoulder Bridge with Leg Lift

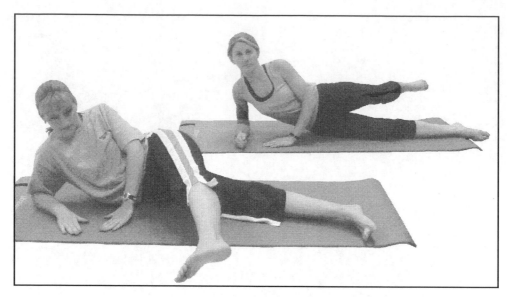

Figure 7.6: Front and Back Leg Kicks

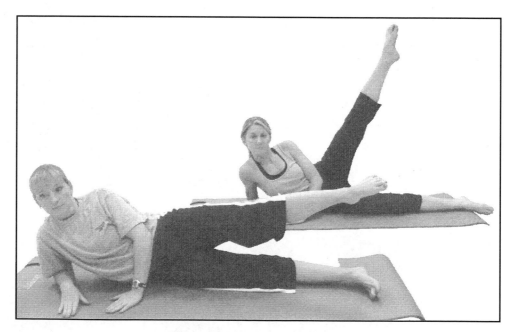

Figure 7.7: Single Leg Raises

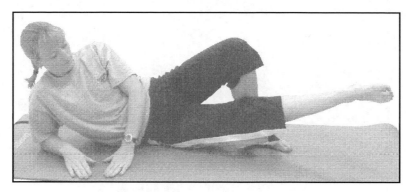

Figure 7.8: Inner Leg Lifts with Leg Behind

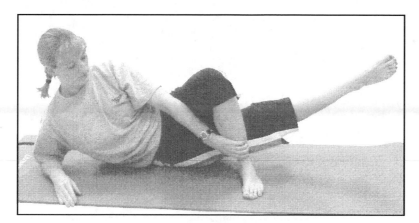

Figure 7.9: Inner Leg Lifts with Leg Front

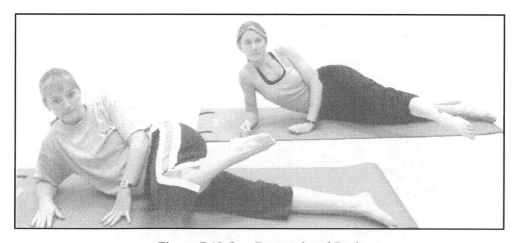

Figure 7.10: Leg Forward and Back

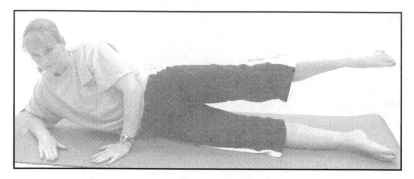

Figure 7.11: Small Leg Circles

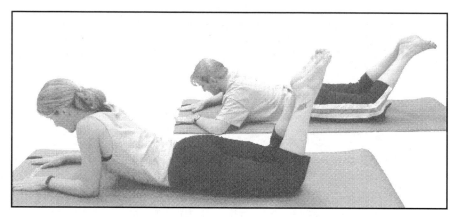

Figure 7.12: Heel Beats and Advanced Heel Beats

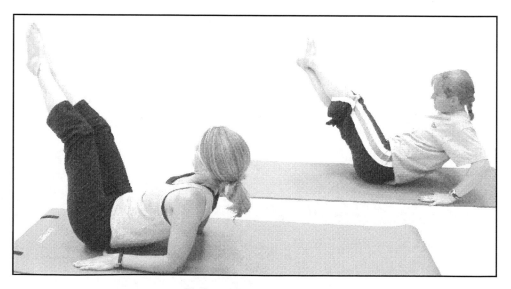

Figure 7.13: Hip Circles

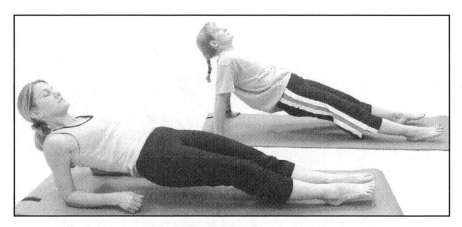

Figure 7.14: Beginning and Advanced Arm Reverse Plank

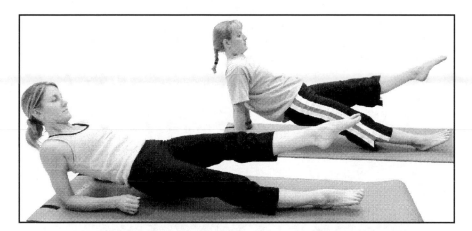

Figure 7.15: Beginning and Advanced Reverse Plank with Leg Lift

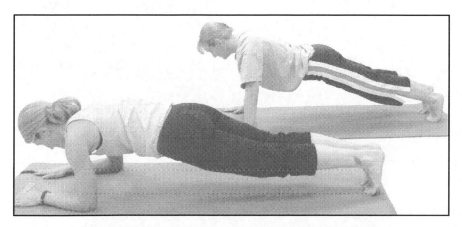

Figure 7.16: Beginning and Advanced Prone Plank

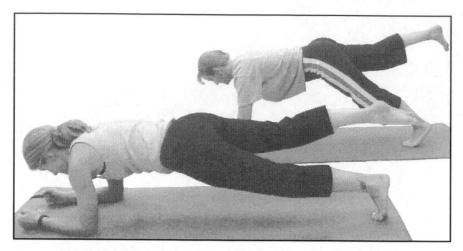

Figure 7.17: Beginning and Advanced Prone Plank with Leg Lift

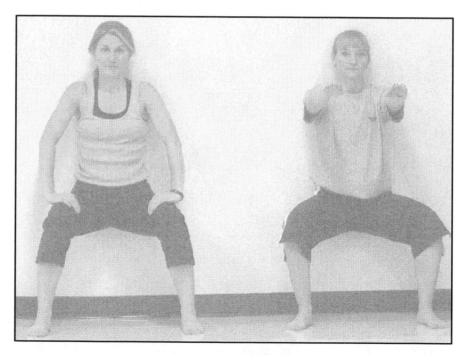

Figure 7.18: Wall Sit

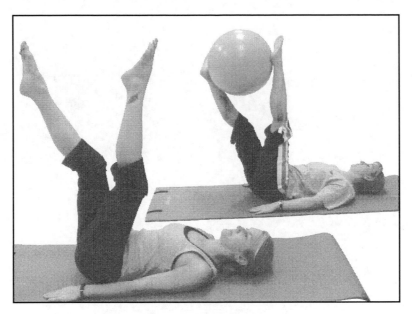

Figure 7.19: Helicopter

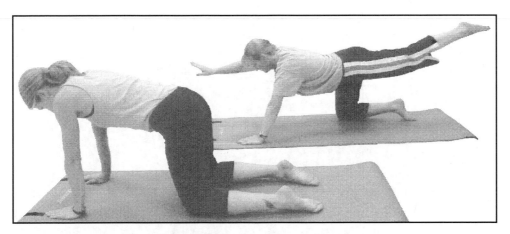

Figure 7.20: Alternating One Arm Superman

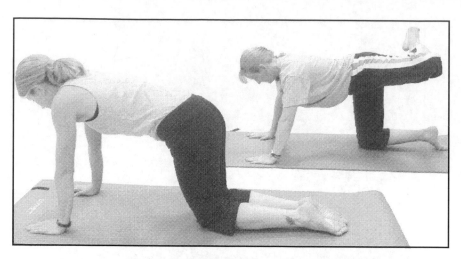

Figure 7.21: Fire Hydrant Leg Lifts

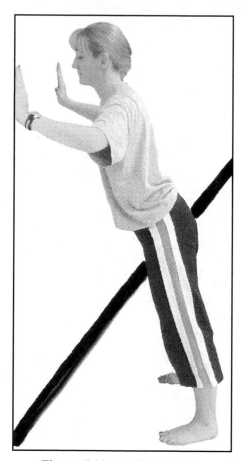

Figure 7.22: Wall Push-ups

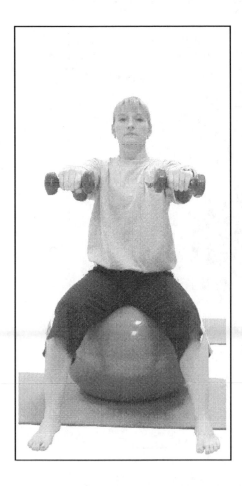

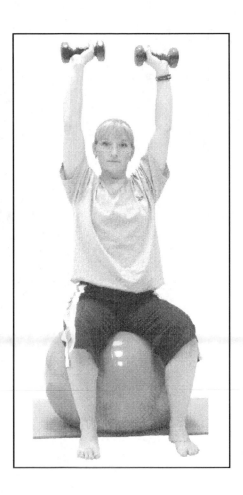

Figure 7.23: Front Arm Raises   **Figure 7.24: Shoulder Press**

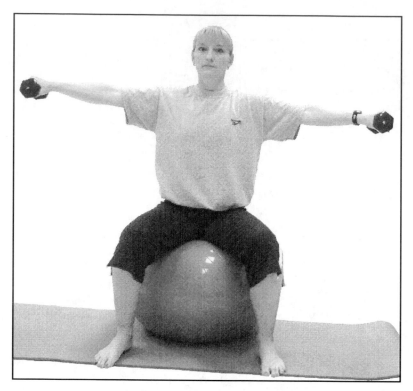

Figure 7.25: Side Arm Raises

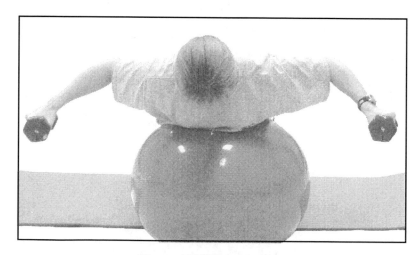

Figure 7.26: Inverse Flys

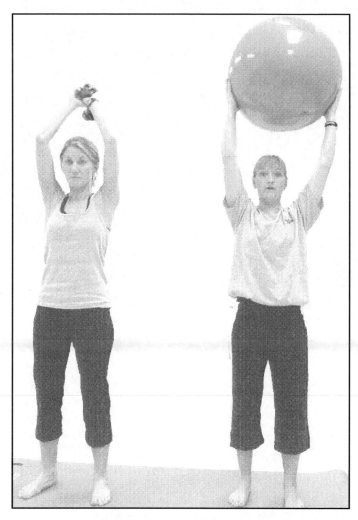

Figure 7.27: Triceps Dip

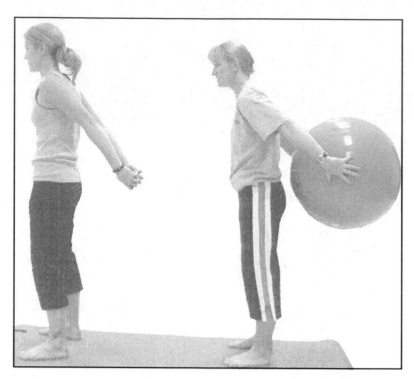

Figure 7.28: Triceps Raises

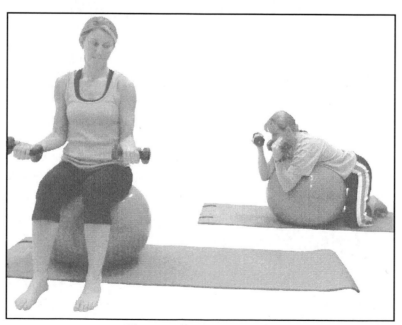

Figure 7.29: Biceps Curls

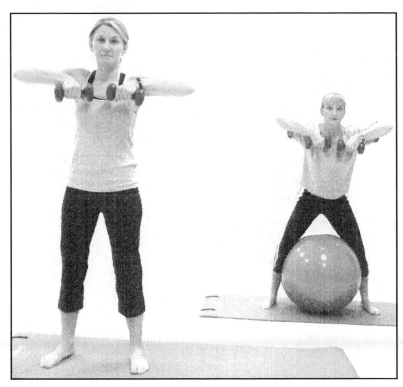

Figure 7.30: Up-Right Rowing

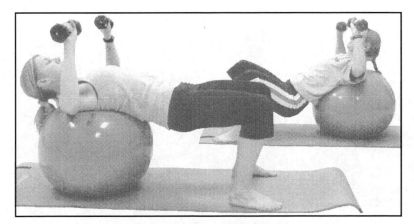

Figure 7.31: Bench Press

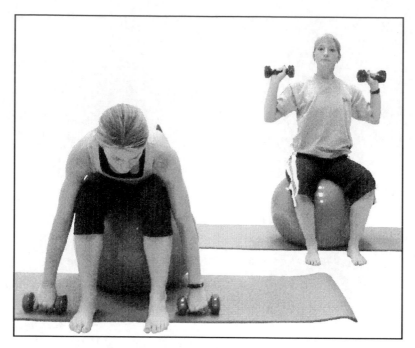

Figure 7.32: Power Clings

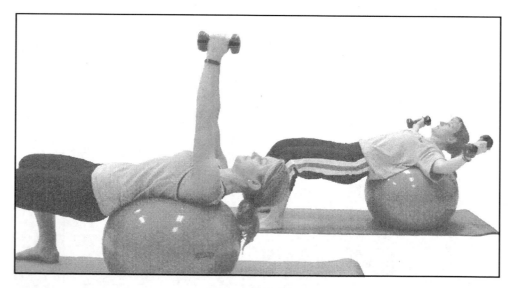

Figure 7.33: Flys

Chapter Eight
STRETCHES

Stretching is an important part of any workout and should be performed when the muscles are warm, limber, and have the ability to lengthen without force or strain. The recommended form of stretching is static rather than ballistic. Static stretching consists of slow sustained lengthening (without bouncing) of a muscle group to increase flexibility (**R**ange **O**f **M**otion), and mobility within the back, torso, neck, arms and legs. A stretch should be held for 20-30 seconds for maximal lengthening.

Stretching can also be a relaxing and stress relieving activity that many people enjoy. In addition to increasing the body's ROM, stretching has shown positive results in reducing the risk of injury as the body is able to withstand impact by absorbing and relieving the shock and force from the joints and bones during exercise (Menezes, 2000).

Pilates exercises incorporate stretching, in addition to gaining strength and muscular tone, simply by performing many of the maneuvers. This will make everyday tasks such as bending, reaching and balancing easier to perform throughout life (Kelly, 2001).

The following are examples of Pilates-based stretches including demonstrations of proper form and technique.

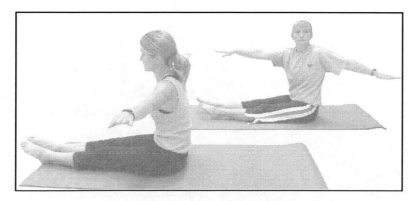

Figure 8.1: Spine Twists

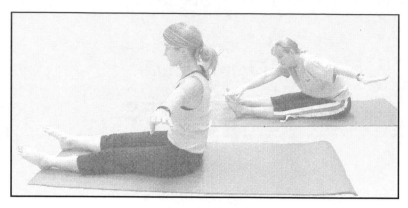

Figure 8.2: Saw

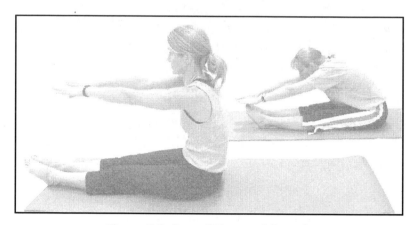

Figure 8.3: Seated Forward Stretch

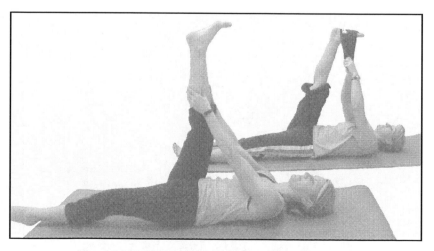

Figure 8.4: Hamstring Stretch and with Towel

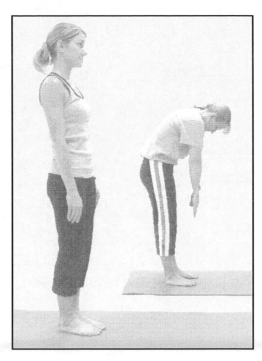

Figure 8.5: Standing Spine Stretch

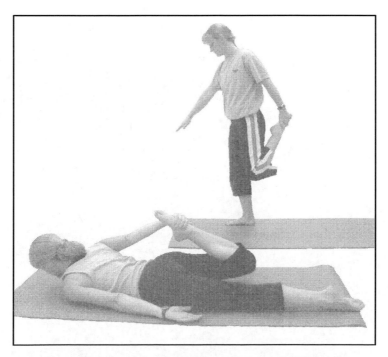

Figure 8.6: Standing and Prone Quadriceps Stretch

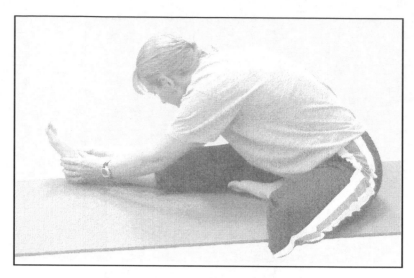

Figure 8.7: Seated Hamstring Stretch

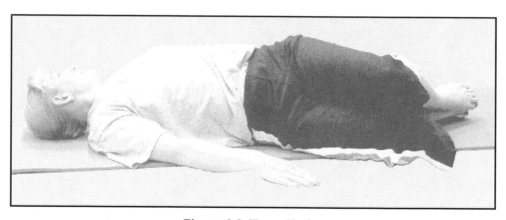

Figure 8.8: Torso Twist

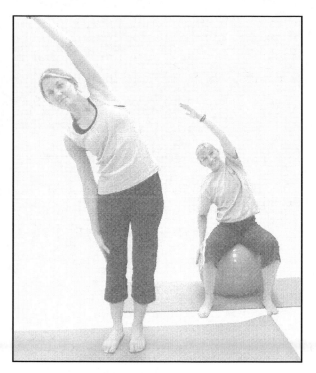

Figure 8.9: Side Bend

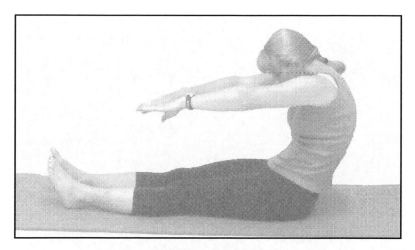

Figure 8.10: Seated "C" Curve

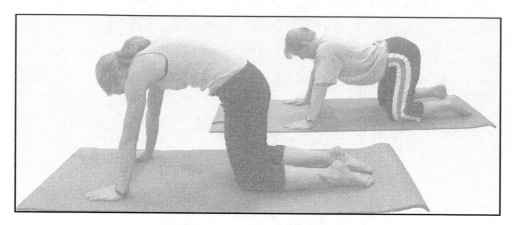

Figure 8.11: Cat Back Stretch

Chapter Nine

PILATES ON THE BALL

Pilates exercises can be performed on a standard exercise ball (55-65 cm in size) which can be purchased just about anywhere today. When choosing the right size ball, a general rule of thumb to follow is that sitting on the ball should make a right angle with legs bent at the knee and feet flat on the floor (Craig, 2003). *Note: A yoga floor mat is suggested to be used during these exercises for safety and comfort.* The ball was originally used for patients in the areas of physical therapy, rehabilitation and orthopedic therapy. The most recent uses of the ball are for physical training of athletes and individuals seeking to improve muscle tone and endurance (Craig, 2003). The exercise ball is inexpensive and easy to learn how to use.

Pilates on the ball is easy to incorporate into a traditional mat Pilates exercise program after having learned the proper form, technique and control. The same guidelines apply to both mat and ball workouts. However, the balance that is required for ball workouts takes some getting used to. In addition, adding the ball exercises to a workout will "spice up" the mat workout and prevent boredom with the same exercises day after day. If you have gotten bored, chances are your muscles have also. Refreshing a workout by adding a ball can increase the amount of exertion the muscles put forth.

Ball Pilates has exercises that will target your arms, chest, legs, back, and gluteus muscles in addition to the "Powerhouse" much like mat Pilates. The following is a list of some exercises for each of the muscle groups that can be used in a Pilates-based workout. Exercises may be performed with or without hand weights to accommodate different fitness levels, beginning with light weights and progressing to heavier as the program continues.

WARM-UP EXERCISES

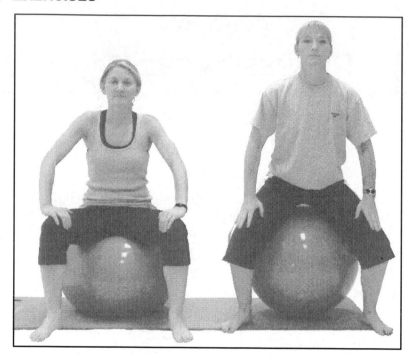

Figure 9.1: Seated Bounce

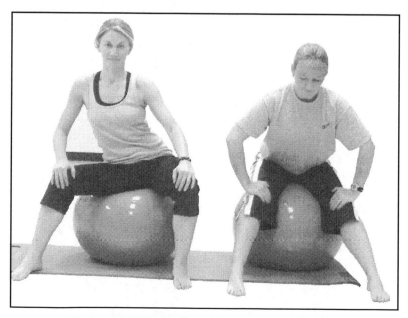

Figure 9.2: Hip Roll: Side to Side; Front/Back

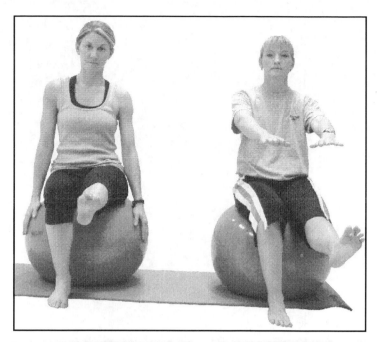

Figure 9.3: Seated Leg Kicks/Extensions

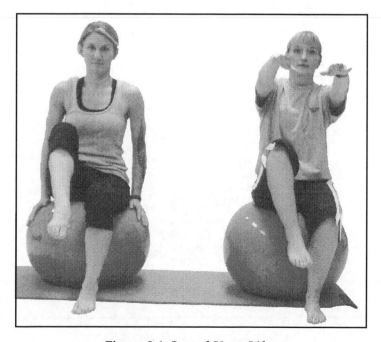

Figure 9.4: Seated Knee Lifts

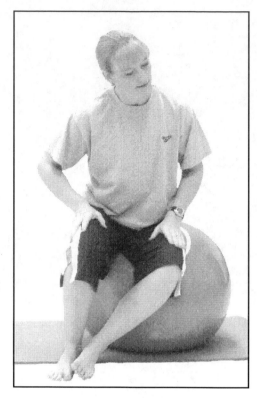

Figure 9.5: Seated Side-to-Side Step

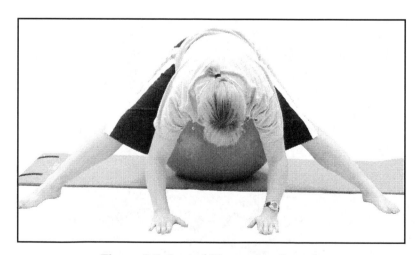

Figure 9.6: Seated Hamstring Stretch

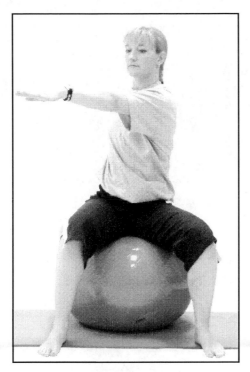

Figure 9.7: Seated Torso Twist

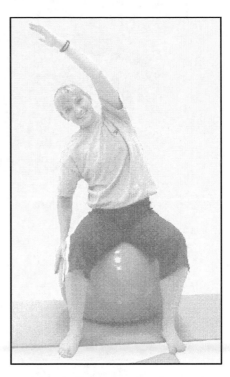

Figure 9.8: Seated Side Bend

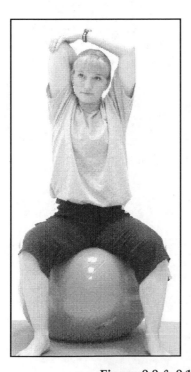

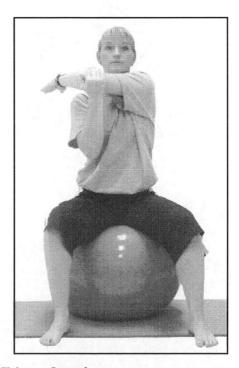

Figure 9.9 & 9.10: Seated Triceps Stretches

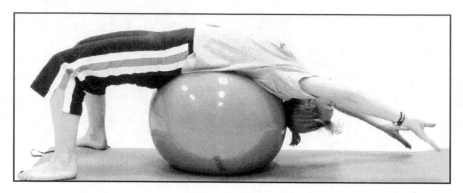

Figure 9.11: Lying Spinal Stretch

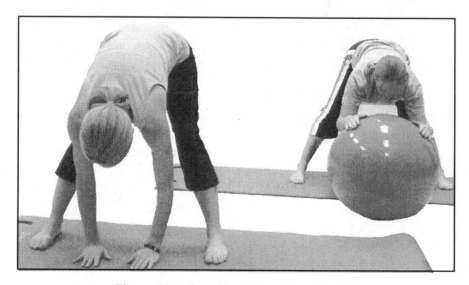

Figure 9.12: Standing Hamstring Stretch

ARM EXERCISES

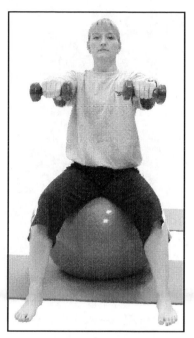

Figure 9.13: Seated Front Arm Raises

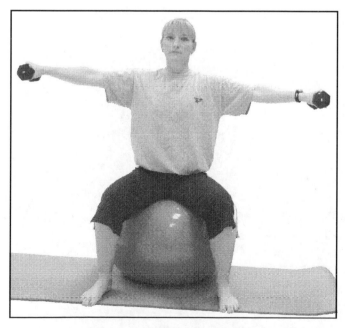

Figure 9.14: Side Arm Raises

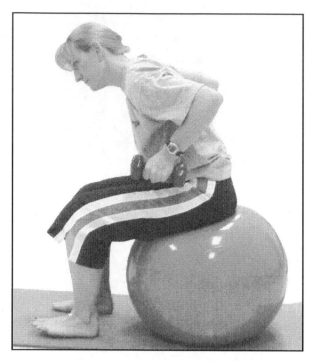

Figure 9.15: Seated Inverse Fly

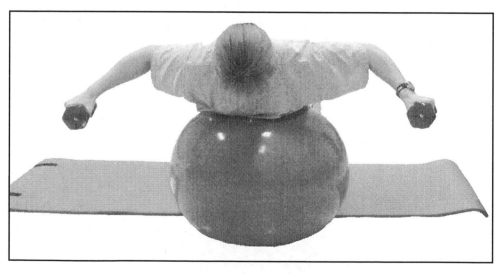

Figure 9.16: Lying Inverse Fly

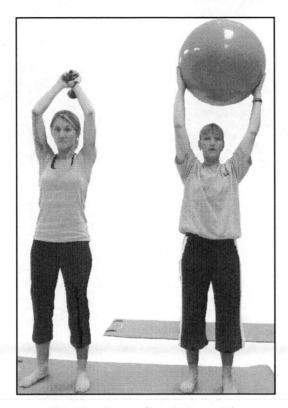

Figure 9.17: Standing Triceps Dips

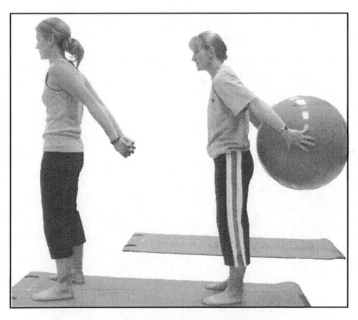

Figure 9.18: Standing Triceps Lifts

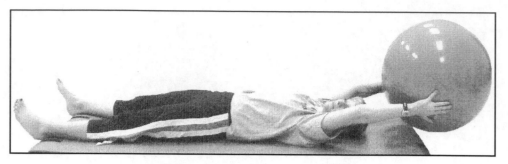

Figure 9.19: Lying Triceps Pumps

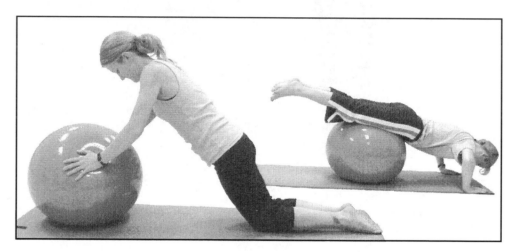

Figure 9.20: Ball Push-ups

LEG EXERCISES

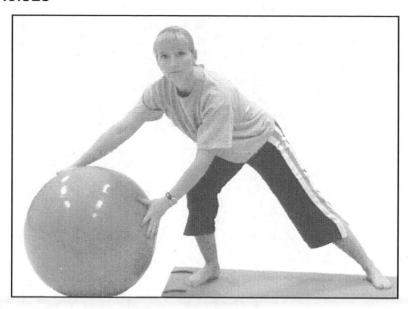

Figure 9.21: Side Lunge & Tap

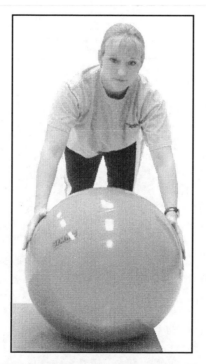

Figure 9.22: Forward Lunge & Tap

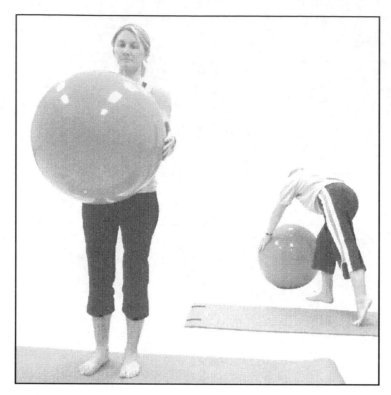

Figure 9.23: Pivot Reverse Lunge & Tap

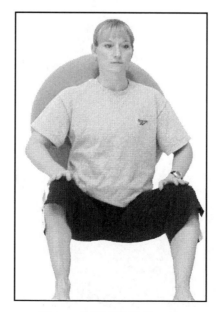

Figure 9.24: Wall Squats

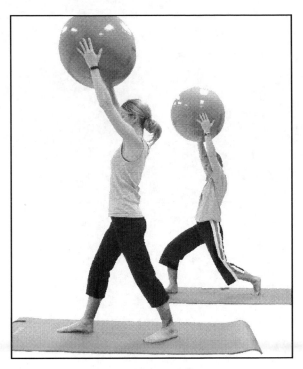

Figure 9.25: Staggerd Leg Squat

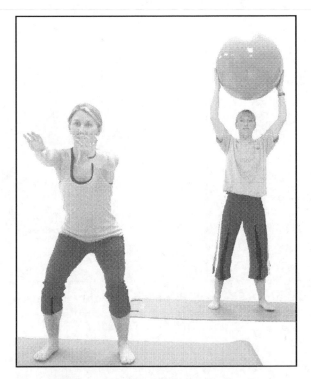

Figure 9.26: Standing Front Squat

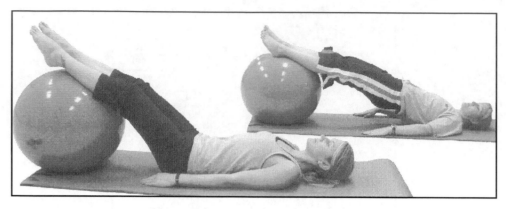

Figure 9.27: Hamstring Press/Lifts

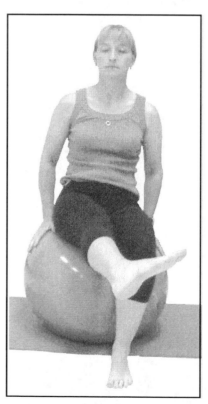
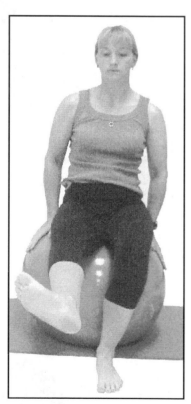

Figures 9.28 and 9.29: Seated Straight Leg Raises
(Toe Inward / Toe Outward)

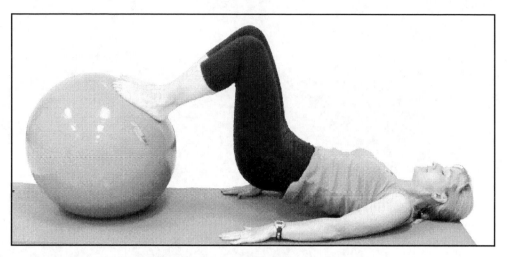

Figure 9.30: Lying Hamstring Rolls

GLUTEUS EXERCISES

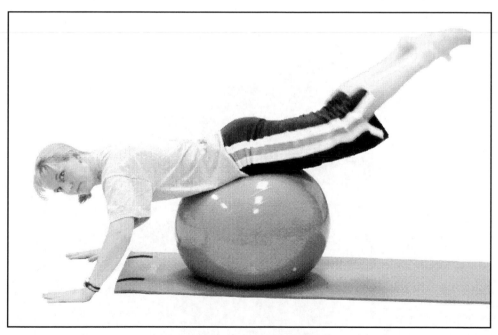

Figure 9.31: Lying Glute Lifts

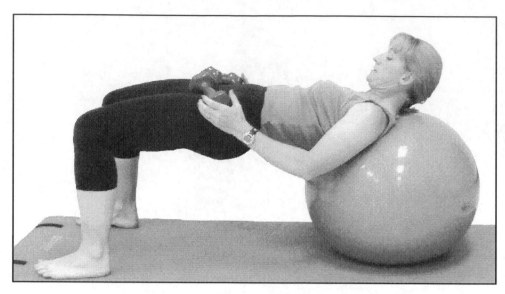

Figure 9.32: Hip Bridge

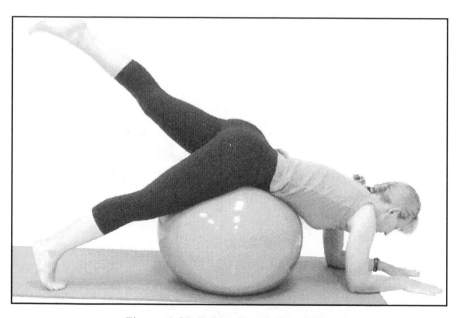

Figure 9.33: Lying Single Leg Lifts

CORE EXERCISES

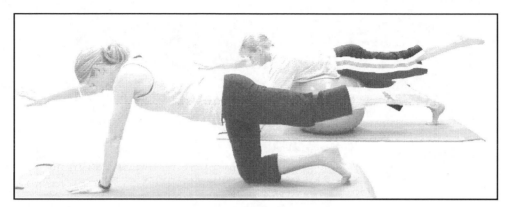

Figure 9.34: One-Arm Superman

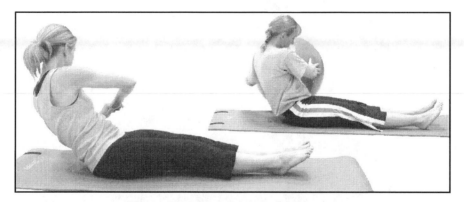

Figure 9.35: Seated Side-to-Side Tap

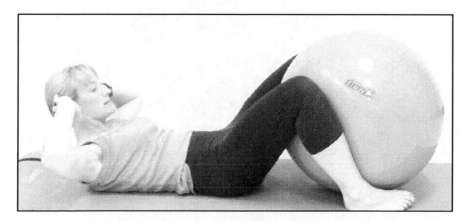

Figure 9.36: Standard Crunch—Ball Squeeze with Knees

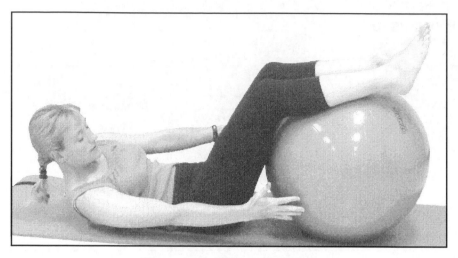

Figure 9.37: Oblique Ball Tap

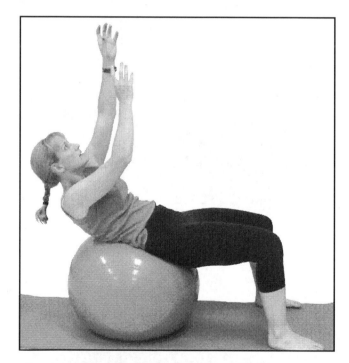

Figure 9.38: Lying Rope Climb

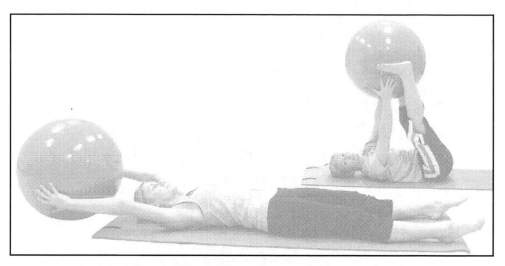

Figure 9.39: Lying Ball Pass and Tap

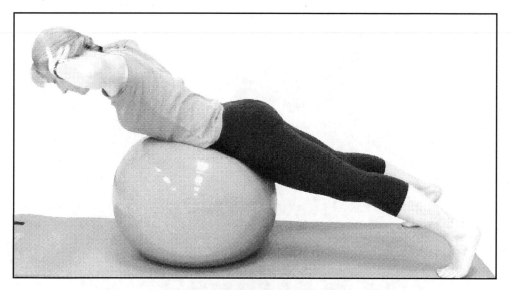

Figure 9.40: Reverse Crunch

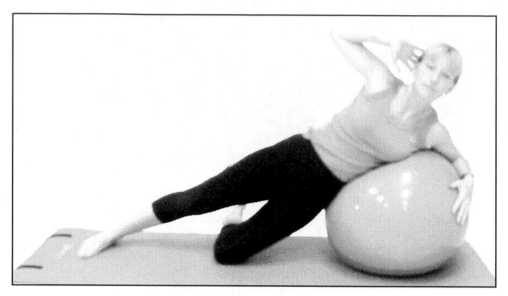

Figure 9.41: Oblique Crunches (version 1)

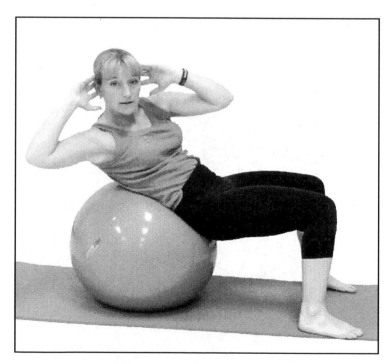

Figure 9.42: Oblique Crunch (version 2)

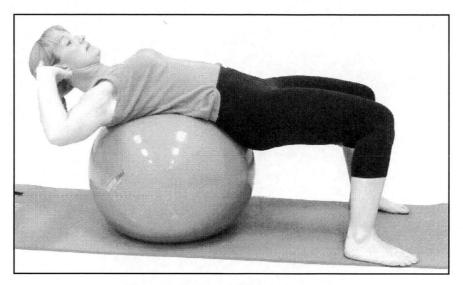

Figure 9.43: Standard Lying Crunch

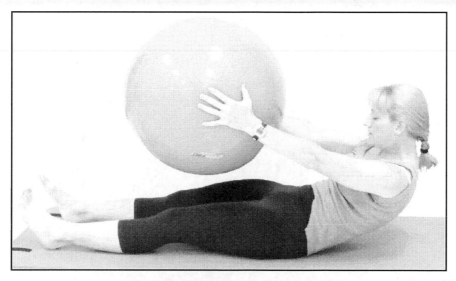

Figure 9.44: The Roll Up with Ball

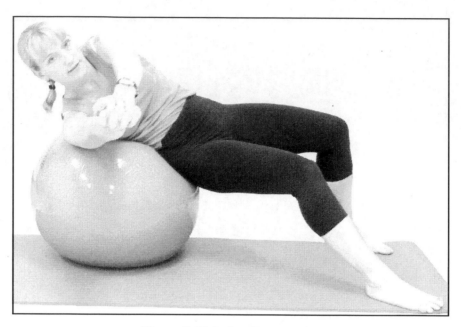

Figure 9.45: Lying Boomerang

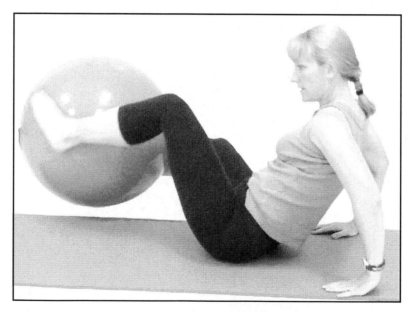

Figure 9.46: Can-Can with Ball

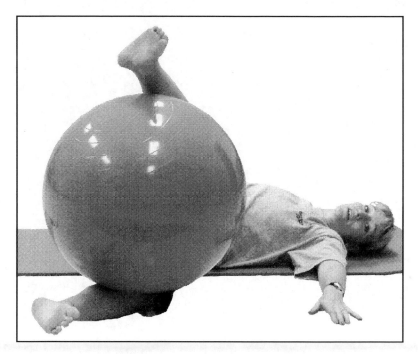

Figure 9.47: Pendulum with Ball

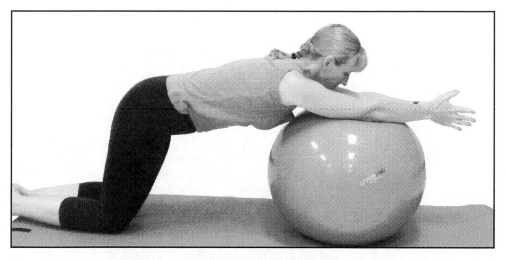

Figure 9.48: Kneeling Roll-out Plank

Chapter Ten
PILATES CIRCUIT WORKOUTS

Circuit workouts consist of several exercise stations. The person performing the exercises (in a class setting or on his own in the living room) rotates through the circuit spending the same amount of time at each station. The goal is to perform the specified Pilates-based exercise for the entire amount of time at that station and move to the next station with little or no rest. This type of workout targets muscular endurance. Each station is allotted the same amount of time which may vary according to the type of workout and the fitness levels of the participants. An average of two to three minutes per station is considered the optimal time because this allows for moving from station to station and getting into position. Circuit workouts may be set up with several stations targeting the same muscle groups back-to-back for a more advanced circuit or one that alternates the major muscle groups from station-to-station for beginning to intermediate levels. The number of stations may also vary depending on the space available, the number of participants, the number of times the circuit will be repeated, the amount of equipment available, and the time allotted for the class. All the Pilates-based exercises that are included in the circuit should have been performed in the regular class setting to ensure that the students are familiar with each one. Once the basic exercises have been learned, a Pilates-based circuit will be fun and easy to implement into the class format.

There are several benefits to using a Pilates-based circuit workout from an instructor's standpoint as well as the participant. Most of the stations require only a mat and the station's instructions for each specific exercise; therefore, if other equipment such as balls and weights are limited, only a few would be required. This would allow all participants the opportunity to use the equipment in a circuit workout which might not be possible in a regular class setting. It takes very little time to set up the circuit because there is very little equipment involved. This benefits both the instructor and student as the workout can become "short and sweet." Once the circuit has been learned and performed by the class, participants automatically know what to expect for the day. Pilates-based circuit workouts have proven to be time efficient and allows for any late arrivals to begin immediately at one of the vacant mats with very little disruption to the rest of the class. The instructor will place extra mats at each station for any participant who may arrive late because it is important that the sequence be followed (warm-up/workout/ stretch). Pilates circuit workouts also act as a "refresher" to the standard mat Pilates class or in-home workout that may have become redundant or predictable. Another benefit of the circuit is that it allows the instructor to move around through the circuit and observe each participant's form and technique from a more advantageous angle than during the regular Pilates class format.

The circuit is a great tool to add variety to the class and get people moving around. Because the stations are timed, there will be some sort of signal to indicate moving on to the next station. The most common ways to signal the change are a verbal command, blowing a whistle, ringing a bell or the use of a timer. Music CD's are also available that start and stop the music.

Pilates-based circuit workouts are easy to design and can be customized to specific workout goals or designed to target specific injuries or problems areas. Your instructor may mix and match any of the exercises in the book to create new and different circuit workouts to meet any specific needs and accommodate all fitness levels.

Students who take this course may benefit from learning to set up circuits as they may have the opportunity to teach these exercises in the future as a fitness instructor, a physical education teacher, a YMCA coordinator, or just leading a group of friends in an informal setting. The set up is easy to learn and easy to use. The following are three examples that show some of the many possible ways that Pilates-based circuits might be set up.

Circuit #1 uses standard mat Pilates-based exercises without extra equipment. It consists of a warm-up, basic core and leg exercises, and stretching. This circuit is created to target many muscles groups but none of them back-to back allowing a rest before fatiguing the same muscles again.

Circuit #2 includes the exercise ball. It also includes a warm-up, core and leg exercises, stretching and adds the element of balance through stabilization. This circuit also alternates major muscle groups.

Circuit #3 is a combination of mat and ball exercises. The stations may alternate the use of a ball or just a mat to keep a variety of exercises in the workout.

REGULAR MAT PILATES: CIRCUIT # 1

- 2 minutes at each station
- Equipment: mat per person per station (1 to 5 participants per station depending on class size)

Warm-up Stations   *Targeted Muscle Group*

#1	The 100 (figure 5.1)	Core
#2	The roll up (figures 5.5 and 5.6)	Core
#3	Straight leg scissors (figure 5.8)	Hamstrings
#4	Leg sweeps (balancing) (figure 5.15)	Gluteus muscles
#5	Pliés (figure 5.12)	Quadriceps/Hamstrings

Workout Stations   *Targeted Muscle Group*

#6	Bicycle (laying on back) (figure 6.1)	Core
#7	Swimmer (figure 6.2)	Low back/Gluteus
#8	Shoulder bridge raises (figure 7.3)	Hamstrings/Gluteus
#9	Single leg raises (figure 7.7)	Abductor muscles
#10	Wall sit (figure 7.18)	Quadriceps
#11	One-armed superman (balancing) (figure 7.20)	Low back/Gluteus
#12	Double leg raise/lower (figure 6.5)	Core
#13	Wall push-ups (figure 7.22)	Upper body

Stretching Stations   *Targeted Muscle Group*

#14	Seated hamstring stretch (figure 9.13)	Hamstrings
#15	Cat back stretch (figure 5.14)	Back / Abdominals
#16	Torso Twist (figure 5.9)	Core
#17	Standing quadriceps stretch (figure 8.6)	Quadriceps

BALL PILATES: CIRCUIT # 2

- 2 minutes per station
- Equipment: 1 mat and 1 ball per person per station

Warm-up Stations

#1	Hip Roll on ball (figure 9.2)
#2	Seated bounce (figure 9.1)
#3	Seated leg extensions (figure 9.3)
#4	Seated knee lifts (figure 9.4)

Workout Stations   *Targeted Muscle Group*

#5	Boomerang (figure 9.45)	Core
#6	Push-ups (laying on ball hands on floor) (figure 9.20)	Upper body
#7	Seated Side taps (figure 9.35)	Abdominals
#8	Side lung/ ball tap (figure 9.21)	Abductor muscles
#9	One armed Superman on ball (balance)(figure 9.34)	Low back/Gluteus
#10	Backwards Triceps Press (arms behind)(figure 9.18)	Triceps
#11	Wall squats with ball (figure 9.24)	Quadriceps
#12	Lying Ball pass and tap (figure 9.39)	Abdominals
#13	Pendulum (figure 9.47)	Adductor muscles

Stretching Stations   *Targeted Muscle Group*

#14	Seated side bend (figure 9.8)	External Obliques
#15	Spinal stretch (laying on top of ball) (figure 9.11)	Back
#16	Seated hamstring stretch (figure 9.6)	Hamstring

COMBINATION CIRCUIT: CIRCUIT # 3

- 2 minutes at each station
- Equipment: 1 mat per person per station, ball at designated stations, small hand weights at designated stations

Warm-up Stations   *Targeted Muscle Group*

	#		
	#1	Single leg pumps (figure 5.2)	Core, Hamstrings
	#2	Roll like a ball (figure 5.7)	Core, Spine
	#3	Can-can (figure 5.11)	Core
Ball	#4	Bounce step side to side (figure 9.5)	Lower body

Workout Stations   *Targeted Muscle Group*

	#		
	#5	Blooming Flower (figure 6.7)	Abdominals
Ball	#6	Standing staggered leg squat (figure 9.25))	Quadriceps, Hamstrings
Ball	#7	Glute lifts (figure 9.31)	Gluteus
Ball + weights	#8	Bicep curls (figure 7.29)	Pectoralis muscles
Ball	#9	Helicopter (figure 9.17)	Abdominals, Adductors
	#10	Heel beats (figure 7.12)	Low back, Hamstrings
Ball	#11	Standing pivot reverse lung w/tap (figure 9.23)	Core, Upper Body, Hamstrings
	#12	Prone plank (with leg lifts) (figure 7.17)	Core, Upper Body, Hamstrings
Ball	#13	Reverse crunch (figure 9.40)	Low Back
	#14	Front and back leg kicks (figure 7.6)	Lower body
Ball + weights	#15	Butterfly arms laying on ball (figure 9.16)	Pectoralis muscles

Stretching Stations   *Targeted Muscle Group*

	#		
Ball	#16	Seated torso twists on ball (figure 9.7)	Upper body, Core
	#17	Lying Prone Quad stretch (figure 8.6)	Quadriceps
Ball + weights	#18	Seated "C" Curve (figure 5.10)	Back
	#19	Seated overhead tricep stretch (figure 9.9)	Triceps
Ball	#20	Seated leg kicks on ball (figure 9.3)	Quadriceps

Chapter Eleven

NUTRITION AND WEIGHT LOSS THE HEALTHY WAY

THE SIX ESSENTIAL NUTRIENTS

Water

Water is a necessary nutrient and is involved in all bodily functions. You can live several weeks without food, but only a few days without water depending on the environment. Don Colbert, M.D. states in his book *The Seven Pillars of Health* that water is the single most important nutrient for our bodies. But many people seem to take water for granted or ignore its importance. To stress the importance of water in bodily functions Dr. Colbert listed the following:

1. The entire body is 70 % water.
2. The muscles are 75% water.
3. The brain cells are 85% water.
4. The blood is 83% water.
5. The bones are 25% water.

Unfortunately most individuals do not drink enough water on a regular basis. It is estimated that a sedentary adult in a controlled (thermoneutral) environment requires 2.5 L of water everyday. If an adult is working in a hot environment the individual's water requirement may increase to between 5 and 10 L daily (McArdle, Katch, & Katch, 2005). Exercise in a hot, humid environment can be very dangerous if fluid replacement is not adequate. Therefore, it is important to replace fluid before you feel thirsty. When an individual exercises, the water lost (through exercise) should be replaced. Our body's thirst mechanism is not extremely efficient and when an individual feels thirsty that individual may already be slightly dehydrated (Colbert, 2007). A person should drink water before, during, and after exercise. It is also recommended to drink approximately eight 8-oz. glasses of water everyday. For individuals who are active this amount should be increased.

Carbohydrates

Carbohydrates are our body's main source of energy and are broken down by the digestion process into glucose. Carbohydrates supply 40-50% of the body's energy when at rest (Cruise, 2005). Carbohydrates are also the preferred fuel for the brain and nervous system (Boyle, Zyla, 1992). When glucose is stored in the muscle or liver it is called glycogen. This is a quick, but limited energy source for our bodies. There are two kinds of carbohydrates: simple and complex. Those that digest quickly are the simple carbohydrates found in milk, fruits, and sweets. Complex carbohydrates are those that take longer to digest and offer longer lasting energy. They include starch and fiber. Starch is found in foods such as bread, rice, and potatoes and fiber is found in plants (Boyle, Zyla, 1992). There are some discrepancies in the percentages of the carbohydrate intake. For many years it has been suggested that carbohydrates should make up 58-60% of our daily diet, but some believe that the percentages should follow the 30-40-30 plan (30% fat, 40% carbohydrates, and 30% protein). Carbohydrates are found in foods such as bread, rice, and potatoes (ACE, 1996). For most individuals carbohydrates should make up 55-60% of our daily diet. Fad diets sometimes eliminate carbohydrates which will result in rapid weight loss. However, when carbohydrates are reintroduced into the diet the weight is regained. This is partially due to water loss not fat loss (ACE, 1996). The body's metabolism may slow due to the lack of energy and carbohydrate intake. This type of high protein- low carbohydrate diet is considered by some to be unhealthy and even dangerous. Fad diets change eating habits for a short period of time and will result in temporary changes. In order for the weight loss changes to be permanent, the eating habits must also be permanent. Unless lifestyle changes in eating habits are made, fad diets are usually unsuccessful, create frustration, and may slow the metabolism. It is best to check with a physician before making any drastic change in dietary habits.

The concept of good carbs. versus bad carbs. has recently become a hot topic. That leaves us with the question, which carbohydrates are good and which carbohydrates are bad? Good carbohydrates include fruits, vegetables, and whole grains. Bad carbohydrates are those that are highly processed and the fiber has been removed (Agatston, 2003). However, it is important to remember that even good carbs have calories and they should not be consumed in excess.

Protein

Proteins are amino acids. The body needs protein to make enzymes and hormones that regulate crucial bodily functions as well as building and repairing body tissue. An adequate protein supply is necessary for health. Protein should make up 10-12% of our daily diet. Protein is found in our body's muscles, organs, antibodies, hormones, and enzymes (Cruise, 2005). It is a misconception to believe that an increased intake of protein will result in a major increase in muscle mass. This is not the case and this excess protein will most likely be stored as fat (McArdle, Katch, & Katch, 2005).

There are two types of protein: complete and incomplete. A source of complete protein will supply all the essential amino acids while an incomplete protein will not. Meat, fish, and poultry are a complete protein source while vegetables, grains, and legumes are considered incomplete because they do not supply the essential amino acids. This is why it is necessary for vegetarians to combine foods properly to provide a complementary protein source due to the absence of meat. By combining certain foods the individual is provided with all the essential amino acids necessary for bodily functions.

Fats (Lipids)

Is fat really the enemy? Fat cushions and surrounds organs for protection. In addition, fat is a secondary source of energy for the body when involved in exercise for a prolonged period of time. Fat should make up 28 – 30% of our diet. Fats can also be referred to as good fats or bad fats. The "bad" fats are the saturated fatty acids. Saturated fats come from animal products and are solid at room temperature. Examples include lard, shortening, and butter. The "good" fats are the unsaturated fatty acids and come primarily from plant source. Examples include corn oil, vegetable oil, and olive oil.

Coronary heart disease is a major health concern today that is why it is important to monitor the level of triglycerides. Triglycerides are the fat that clogs arteries (Agatston, 2003). Triglycerides are the chemical form in which most fat whether in the body or in food exists. Regardless to the type of food that you eat any calories that are ingested during a meal and not used immediately will be converted to triglycerides (American Heart Association, 2007). Obese people have uncontrolled diabetes, hypothyrodism, kidney disease, and individuals with a family history of high triglycerides are more likely to have high triglycerides (WebMD, 2007). Therefore, it is important to limit the intake of triglycerides by eating more unsaturated fats.

Vitamins

Vitamins (organic substances) do not provide fuel for the body, but they are needed for energy production as well as growth and bodily repair (ACE, 1996). Eating a balanced diet should provide necessary vitamins needed for general health. However, the majority of people today do not get an adequate source of vitamins by diet alone due to the way foods are processed, the way foods are cooked, and poor eating habits. Vitamins are not needed in great quantities, therefore; it is important not to fall victim to the "more is better" way of thinking. Many people read about the benefits of certain vitamins and think that if a little is good then more would be better. This can be a fatal mistake. Vitamins are either water soluble (all the B Vitamins and Vitamin C) or fat soluble (Vitamins A, D, E, and K). Vitamins that are fat soluble can accumulate in the body and have a toxic affect.

Most agree that there is little danger in taking a multi-vitamin and that vitamin supplementation may offer benefits to physically active individuals, particularly those who have marginal vitamin stores available and those who do not eat a proper diet. Further research in this area is still needed to determine just how significant these benefits are (McArdle, Katch & Katch, 2007).

Minerals

Minerals (inorganic substances) also do not provide fuel for the body, but are necessary for vital bodily functions. Minerals are important in the regulation of the heart beat, building bones and teeth, oxygen transportation to cells, formation of hemoglobin, and in muscle contraction. Minerals are divided into two categories according to the amount that is needed: major and minor (trace). Major minerals include calcium, phosphorous, sodium, chloride, and magnesium. Minor minerals include iron, zinc, copper, iodine, manganese, molybdenum, arsenic, boron, nickel and silicon (ACE, 1996).

Most diets provide an adequate source of minerals with the exception of calcium and iron. The lack of calcium and iron is usually seen in women (McArdle, Katch, & Katch, 2007).

HEALTHY EATING FOR OPTIMAL WEIGHT

Three of the six essential nutrients provide calories for the body. They are carbohydrates, proteins, and fats. Each gram of carbohydrate and protein provides four calories and each gram of fat provides nine calories. (FYI: alcohol provides seven calories per gram.) The other three essential nutrients, water, minerals and vitamins are necessary for our bodily functions.

A balanced diet will include all of the six essential nutrients necessary for optimal health. The key to good nutrition is being a wise consumer and being able to make educated decisions regarding healthy eating habits. Reading food labels is one way to know exactly what is being consumed. Manufacturer food labels are required to provide basic product information to the consumer such as quantity of contents, list of ingredients in descending order, nutrient values (fat, sodium, fiber, sugar, cholesterol, etc.) and calorie content. This makes it easier to determine what is healthy food and what is not. However, if food nutritional value is not a top priority in food selection compared to taste or cost value, a person may not consult the food label for nutritional facts (Guthrie, Derby & Levy).

Fast foods are not the best choice when trying to eat a healthy balanced diet especially if you are trying to lose weight. Eating trends of Americans today have become a great deal of the problem in our overall health. People are eating more fast food than ever due to lack of time to cook at home and lifestyles on the run. Food consumed away from home typically contains more fat, saturated fat, and cholesterol compared to those cooked at home (Kennedy, Blaylock & Kuhn). Because people are eating out more the food is primarily cooked with saturated fats, deep fried and greasy. It's easy to go to McDonalds and feed a family of four for under $10 with the $1.00 menu; however it is not the healthiest choice. Some eating establishments offer a heart healthy section or low-fat entrees on their menus for those who are making a conscious effort to eat healthy. You may be able to get a healthier meal by substituting certain side dishes; for example, ask for a baked potato or a side salad instead of french fries. Another example of healthy substituting is to drink water with meals rather than tea or sodas to eliminate unnecessary sugar and calories. For example, in 1977 the consumption of cokes was about half as much as milk or coffee and in 1995 the consumption of cokes increased 130%. Consumption of many high sugar–added foods increased during the last decade (Tippett & Cleveland). Portion control also plays a role in Americans unhealthy eating trends. Portions are much larger than they used to be, both at home and at restaurants. "American consumers have lost sight of a proper portion size and that's not hard to do in our "bigger is better" society; portion sizes in most restaurants and throughout the grocery stores are geared towards lumberjacks," states Professor Judith Stern. Portion control is compromised when all-you-can-eat buffet style restaurants are becoming more and more common. Americans' have the idea that there is a need to get our money's worth; therefore, we eat much more than we would otherwise. Restaurants are using this concept to draw customers in by offering to Super Size the fries and coke for just $.39 extra. We can't refuse. The single portion sizes being served at most restaurants today could easily feed two people.

Our bodies are magnificent creations that were designed to survive. The storage of fat was necessary for survival during times of famine. Due to technology and modernization we have become a society that values leisure time and continues to search for ways to reduce physical labor which leads to sedentary lifestyles that contribute to obesity and other health-related conditions. Obesity is a major health concern today. It is reported that the obesity rate among children is on the rise. A sad fact is that once a child becomes over-weight, that child will most likely be an over-weight adult. Research has shown that one of the side effects of obesity is insulin resistance. Diabetes is the condition where the hormone insulin is unable to properly process carbohydrates and fats. This condition causes the body to store more fat particularly in the midsection (Agatston, 2003). Insulin resistance could cause cardiovascular troubles in the future.

NUTRITION TIPS

- Don't cut too many calories at once during weight loss, reduce slowly so the body can adjust metabolism
- Don't fear fat, moderation is the key
- Eat high calorie/high carb. meals early in the day, more time to burn them off
- Reduce salt intake if bloating occurs, results in water retention
- Eat breakfast to jump start your metabolism
- Go grocery shopping on a full stomach, it reduces impulse buying
- Cut back on cocktails, they contain a great deal of calories
- Track improvements by body fat% or the way clothes fit (loose/tight), NOT only scale weight (muscle weighs more)
- Weigh in the morning no more than once per week (same time, same scale, same conditions)
- Successful weight loss is 1-2 lbs. per week
- Always include physical activity with diet (healthy eating) when attempting weight loss (diet alone can result in loss of lean mass)
- Avoid late night meals or snacks to avoid becoming stored as fat
- Snacks should be approximately 100 calories or less
- Eating 5-7 times per day sustains the metabolism (less than 3 meals per day slows the metabolism)

BASAL METABOLIC RATE (BMR)

Basal Metabolic Rate (BMR) contributes to the amount of calories burned and is defined as the number of calories used to sustain life such as breathing, digestion, heart beat, and lung expansion. This calorie burning takes place within the body and is involuntary. The formula to calculate BMR is as follows:

1. Figure body weight in kilograms (number of lbs. divided by 2.2)
2. Multiply weight in kilograms by .90 (which is hourly calories burned)
3. Multiply results above by 24 for the number of calories burned per day (24 hour period)

This equation will provide an approximate daily BMR. Add the calories burned from exercise to the BMR to estimate the number of calories expended in a 24-hour period. For example, a 145 lb. woman needs to take in 1,423 calories per day just to stay alive. According to nutrition labels, the average caloric intake is 2,000 per day; however, many Americans consume many more calories than are expended. The average daily caloric intake in 1994 was 2,002 kcal compared to 1,854 in 1978. Today the caloric intake is rarely under 2,500 per day. To stay the same body weight, people must balance the calories consumed and the calories used by the body (food energy). Physical activity is an important component in burning those calories and maintaining that balance (Tippett & Cleveland). Regular physical activity is recognized as a way to reduce the risk of becoming overweight as well as developing heart disease in adults and children (Crane, Hubbard & Lewis).

THE FOOD GUIDE PYRAMID

The first USDA (United States Department of Agriculture) food guide was developed in 1916 and has been revised many times since to adapt according to the advances in nutritional knowledge and changes in dietary needs. In the mid 1980's a revised version was developed and released in 1992 and became known as the Food Guide Pyramid because of its graphic representation of the suggested daily recommended servings of each of the six food groups (Guthrie, Derby & Levy). If followed, the Pyramid offers a well balanced diet with variety, moderation and portion control. Although, following a healthy diet is much like trying to balance a teeter-totter because it is easier to eat the "wrong" foods. Today's society associates the order of importance from top to bottom or big to little. This is why our pyramid is rotated 180 degrees to reflect society's way of thinking. The larger the section is on the Pyramid, the more that food group is needed in the daily diet. The smallest section on the Pyramid suggests that food group is recommended in smaller amounts. This was established to make it easier for the public to translate into everyday use. Although the Food Guide Pyramid has been around for many years many people still are not clear how to use it or choose not take the advice it gives.

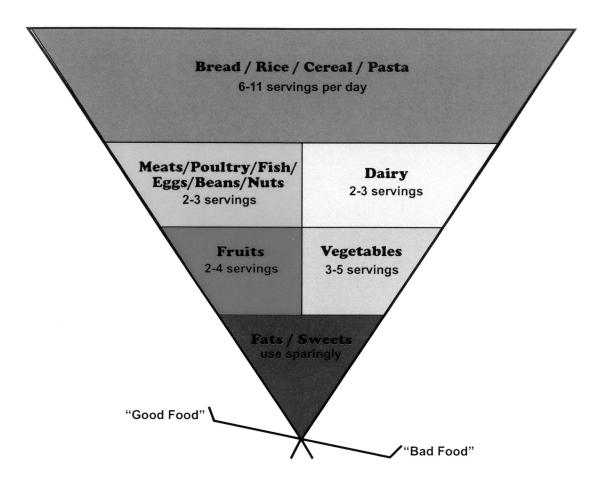

Chapter Twelve
EXERCISE MISCONCEPTIONS

1. Lifting weights will make you bulky like a bodybuilder—F
2. If I'm not sore after a workout, I didn't work hard enough—F
3. I have to sweat profusely to indicate a "good" workout—F
4. Wearing a plastic sweat suit is an effective way to lose weight—F
5. The faster I lift my weights, the more effective I am being—F
6. The longer I am in the weight room or "gym" the better the workout is—F
7. The faster I lose weight the better—F
8. Fad diets will help lose weight AND keep it off—F
9. Changing from regular sodas to diet sodas is healthy—F (Roberts, 1988)
10. Carbs are the enemy—F
11. A soda or candy bar will boost your energy level for a full workout—F (Endurance Marketing Group, 2006)
12. Exercise like Pilates and Yoga are sissy and for girls only—F
13. You must spend high dollar amounts on a gym membership to get results—F
14. Standing on a weight scale tells us how fit we are—F
15. A healthy goal is 0% body fat—F
16. All cardio machines (stationary bike/ elliptical/treadmill/steppers) burn the same amount of calories in a 30 minute workout—F
17. Performing strength training will make you less flexible—F
18. All exercise programs offer the same benefits—F
19. Yo-Yo dieting is not harmful to our bodies—F
20. It is not possible to drink too much water—F
21. Fat will turn into muscle as a result of exercise—F

22. Muscle turns back into fat when exercise is discontinued—F

23. It is possible to reduce fat cells in a particular area of the body by focusing on it during a workout—F

GLOSSARY OF TERMS

Aerobic: "With oxygen", movements or exercises that require continued use of oxygen. Activities typically lasting 20-30+ minutes without break in movement. Examples: swimming, jogging, biking.

Abduction: Movement away from midline of the body.

Adduction: Movement toward the midline of the body.

Alignment: A position of the body where bones and joints are symmetrically in line to avoid strain or injury. Used to create balance.

Anaerobic: "Without oxygen", movements or exercises that use only the oxygen supply that is already available for use without needing additional supplies. Examples: a sprint, a golf swing, strength training.

Ballistic stretching: A form of stretching that incorporates bouncing to lengthen the muscle. No longer the method of choice, may cause damage.

Basal Metabolic Rate (BMR): The amount of calories burned to sustain life (breathing, digestion, heart beating, etc.)

Body Composition: The ratio of lean body mass to fat mass (Men average = 15-18% Women average = 22-25% Over 30% = obese)

Body Mass Index (BMI): A statistical measure in ratio form of scale weight to height (Body weight divided by the square of height).

Contrology: The original term given to the Pilates method due to the use of slow controlled movements and exercises.

Cool-down: The final stage of an exercise bout that is reduced in intensity to allow the pulse to slow and prevent blood pooling. Consists of 3-5 minutes. An example includes riding a stationary bike or walking.

Core: The combination of the abdominal muscles and the back muscles.

Endurance: Muscle's ability to perform and withstand exercises and movements over a prolonged period of time.

Extension: Lengthening or straightening.

Flexibility: The lengthening of a muscle to increase its range of motion.

Flexion: Shortening or bending to bring two body parts closer together.

Health Related Skills: (5 Components of fitness) Cardiovascular endurance (3 minute step test/ 1 mile run/3 mile walk) muscular endurance (1 minute crunch test) muscular strength (1 minute push up test) flexibility (sit and reach/ trunk lift) body composition (bioelectric impedance/skin folds/ hydrostatic weighing).

Holistic approach: The concept of introducing the Pilates method and its easy to learn exercises to people with the hopes that they will individualize a program that suits their needs and abilities.

Hyperextension: extending beyond normal range of motion.

Ligament: attaches bone to bone.

Major minerals: Animals and humans need minerals, including sodium, potassium, calcium, magnesium, and phosphorus in large amounts to regulate and control the normal function of human and animal tissues, muscles, and organs.

Muscular endurance: The muscle's ability to contract repeatedly or to hold a contraction for a period of time.

Muscular strength: The muscle's ability to exert maximal force in a single attempt.

Opposition: Using muscle groups or body parts to perform against another muscle group or body part to add resistance.

Overload: More than normal exercise or intensity accomplished by increasing intensity (difficulty) or time of exercise.

Plank (bridge): A position of the body where muscles are used to support one's own body weight while suspended in air.

Powerhouse: The collective muscles in the abdominals, back, gluteus maximus, and gluteus medias.

Progression: Gradually and systematically increasing the demands on the body.

Prone: Facing the body with stomach side down.

RDA: Recommended Daily Allowance. The recommended amount of certain foods to be taken in on a daily basis that is established by the Food and Nutrition Board of the National Academy of Sciences.

Repetitions: The number of times a specific exercise is performed.

Reversibility: The "use it or lose it" theory that implies that stopping an exercise program will result in benefits gradually being lost.

RICE: Rest, Ice, Compression, Elevate. A common treatment for minor injuries.

ROM: Range of motion around a joint.

Specificity: When the body adapts to the specific type of training.

Spot reducing: A myth that states the body is able to burn fat and tone one specific area of the body.

Static stretching: A slow sustained method of stretching that is held steady that allows the muscle to lengthen slowly.

Supine: Facing the body with back side down.

Tendon: Attaches muscle to bone.

Threshold: The maximal effort possible to expend while performing an exercise.

Trace minerals: Minerals the body needs each day in small amounts for good health. Examples include iron, zinc, copper, selenium, chromium, and iodine.

Valsalva Maneuver: Performing an expiratory effort with a closed mouth and held breath which increases pressure impeding venous blood flow to the heart.

Warm-up: Designed to prepare the body for vigorous exercise beginning with slow, rhythmic activity that gradually increases pace. Consists of 5-10 minutes in length. An example includes walking on a treadmill or riding a stationary bike.

Appendix A

HEALTH FORM

_____ DEPARTMENT

NAME _____ DATE _____

ADDRESS _____

CITY _____ STATE _____ ZIP CODE _____

TELEPHONE # _____ CLASS _____ AGE _____

I. **IF YOU HAVE ANY OF THE FOLLOWING CONDITIONS, PLACE A CHECK IN THE BLANK.**

Disorder	*If yes, check blank.*	*Date*	*Release Date*
A. Anemia	_____	_____	_____
B. Arthritis	_____	_____	_____
C. Asthma	_____	_____	_____
D. Bad Knees	_____	_____	_____
E. Bronchitis (chronic)	_____	_____	_____
F. Cancer	_____	_____	_____
G. Coronary Heart Disease	_____	_____	_____
H. Diabetes	_____	_____	_____
I. Emphysema	_____	_____	_____
J. Epilepsy	_____	_____	_____
K. Heart Attack	_____	_____	_____
L. Heart Surgery	_____	_____	_____
M. High Blood Pressure	_____	_____	_____
N. Kidney Disease	_____	_____	_____
O. Liver Disease	_____	_____	_____
P. Low Back Pain	_____	_____	_____
Q. Rheumatic heart Disease	_____	_____	_____
R. Stroke	_____	_____	_____
S. Ulcer	_____	_____	_____
T. Other	_____	_____	_____
U. Pregnancy	_____	_____	_____

ARE YOU PRESENTLY ON ANY MEDICATION? _____ YES _____ NO

IS THERE ANY HISTORY OF HEART DISEASE IN YOUR FAMILY? _____ YES _____ NO

IS THERE ANY HISTORY OF HEART DISEASE IN YOUR FAMILY? _____ YES _____ NO

ARE YOU CURRENTLY INVOLVED IN ANY EXERCISE PROGRAM? _____ YES _____ NO

DO YOU SMOKE? _____ YES _____ NO

ARE YOU HAPPY WITH YOUR CURRENT WEIGHT? _____ YES _____ NO

ARE YOU CURRENTLY FOLLOWING A SPECIAL DIET? _____ YES _____ NO

WHAT ARE YOUR FEELINGS ABOUT EXERCISE? _____ Enjoyable _____ Boring _____ Other

ARE YOU CURRENTLY UNDER STRESS? _____ Low _____ Moderate _____ High

PRIOR TO WORKOUT, PLEASE READ, COMPLETE, SIGN AND RETURN THIS HEALTH FORM TO YOUR INSTRUCTOR.

* If any above mentioned conditions exist or 1 or more "yes" answers occur a physician should be consulted prior to participation.

NAME _____ DATE _____
                        PLEASE PRINT

YOU MUST HAVE A DOCTOR'S WRITTEN PERMISSION TO ENGAGE IN THIS COLLEGE KINESIOLOGY CLASS IF YOU HAVE ANY OF THE FOLLOWING: DIABETES, HEART PROBLEMS, PREGNANCY, HIGH BLOOD PRESSURE, LUNG PROBLEMS, EXTREMELY OVERWEIGHT, UNDER EXTREME STRESS, OR HAVE HISTORY OF HYPERVENTILATING.

"I, _____ have enrolled in a program of strenuous physical activity including but not limited to aerobic dance, circuit workouts, interval training, jogging, running, stationary cycling, step workouts, weight training activities, and various sport activities. I hereby affirm that I am in good physical condition and do not suffer from any disability that would prevent or limit my participation in this class. I _____ for myself, my heirs and assigns, hereby release the college (its employees and Board of Trustees), from any claims, demands and causes of action arising from my participation in this exercise program and I, _____, hereby release the class instructor from any liability now or in the future including but not limited to heart attacks, muscle strains, pulls or tears, broken bones, shin splints, heat prostration, head, neck, knee, back, or foot injuries and any other illness, soreness or injury however caused, occurring during or after participation in this class."

I HEREBY AFFIRM THAT I HAVE READ AND FULLY UNDERSTAND THE ABOVE.

_____   _____
        SIGNATURE   DATE

Appendix B

GOAL INVENTORY

1. Specific goal I would like to achieve during this class:

2. Reasons why it is important for me to achieve this goal:

    a)
    b)
    c)

3. Name specific outcomes that will result in achieving my goal:

    a)
    b)
    c)

4. Identify the barriers and strategies related to my achieving my goal:

    | *Barriers* | *Strategies* |
    | *(things that hinder me)* | *(ways to overcome the barriers)* |
    | a) | a) |
    | b) | b) |
    | c) | c) |

5. My plan of action to achieve this goal includes doing what:

    a)
    b)
    c)

6. When I am successful I will reward myself by:

7. After achieving this goal I plan to continue these exercise habits for how long _____.

8. In addition to my instructor, I choose _____ as a workout partner to help me stay motivated and achieve my goal.

9. I, _____ (signature) agree to work hard towards achieving this goal by attending class regularly and fully participating in all exercises.

10. The day I choose to begin working on my goal: Today's Date_____

Appendix C

BODY MEASUREMENTS

Name _____ Date_____

Measure the following body areas with a tape measure in inches to determine progress throughout the semester.

Area	Pre	Mid	Post
Body Weight			
Biceps	R L	R L	R L
Chest			
Abdomen			
Hips			
Thighs	R L	R L	R L
Calves	R L	R L	R L

SKINFOLD MEASUREMENTS OR BIOELECTRIC IMPEDANCE RESULTS

Pre Body Composition

Lean Mass _____% = Lean mass Lbs.

Fat _____% = Fat mass Lbs.

Post Body Composition

Lean Mass _____% = Lean mass Lbs.

Fat _____% = Fat mass Lbs.

TARGET HEART RATE

KARVONEN EQUATION

TARGET HEART RATE ZONE CALCULATIONS

Age_____   RHR _____ (Resting Heart Rate)

Beginning	60% – 70%
Intermediate	70% – 80%
Advanced	80% – 85%

Step 1:   220 – _____ = _____ MHR (Estimated Maximum Heart Rate)
                        AGE

Step 2:   _____ – _____ = _____ HRR (Heart Rate Reserve)
                  MHR   RHR

Step 3:   _____ X 60% = _____ + _____ = _____ Low Target Zone
                  HRR   %   RHR

Step 4:   _____ X 85% = _____ + _____ = _____ High Target Zone
                  HRR   %   RHR

Round Off Your Answer
.1 to .4 drop-------.5 to .9 add 1

Target Heart Rate
_____TO_____

TARGET HEART RATE ZONE CALCULATIONS

Age_____   RHR _____ (Resting Heart Rate)

Beginning   60% – 70%
Intermediate   70% – 80%
Advanced   80% – 85%

Step 1:   220 – _____ = _____ MHR (Estimated Maximum Heart Rate)
                    AGE

Step 2:   _____ – _____ = _____ HRR (Heart Rate Reserve)
              MHR   RHR

Step 3:   _____ X 60% = _____ + _____ = _____ Low Target Zone
              HRR   %   RHR

Step 4:   _____ X 85% = _____ + _____ = _____ High Target Zone
              HRR   %   RHR

Round Off Your Answer
.1 to .4 drop-------.5 to .9 add 1

Target Heart Rate
_____TO_____

4-DAY NUTRITION LOG

Day #1	Food	Calorie Count
Breakfast		
Lunch		
Dinner		
Snacks		
Total Sum of Daily Calories:		

Day #2	Food	Calorie Count
Breakfast		
Lunch		
Dinner		
Snacks		
Total Sum of Daily Calories:		

Day #3	Food	Calorie Count
Breakfast		
Lunch		
Dinner		
Snacks		
Total Sum of Daily Calories:		

Day #4	Food	Calorie Count
Breakfast		
Lunch		
Dinner		
Snacks		
Total Sum of Daily Calories:		

Appendix F

MUSCLE DIAGRAMS

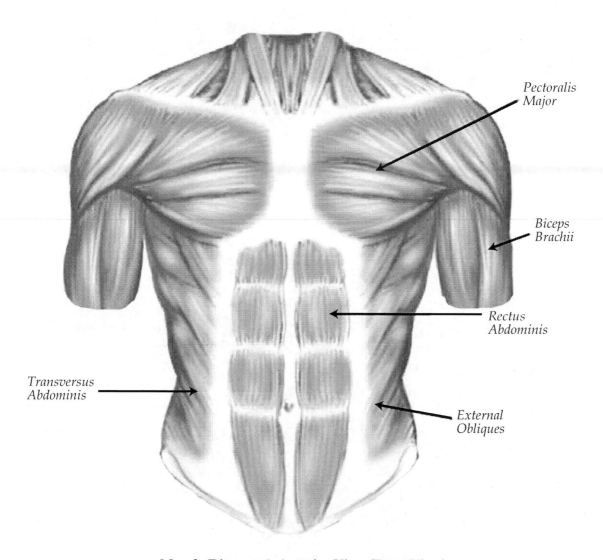

Muscle Diagram 1. Anterior View (Front View)
[adapted from http://bsdweb.bsdvt.org/~aarchacki/pdfs/Muscle%20Diagrams.pdf]

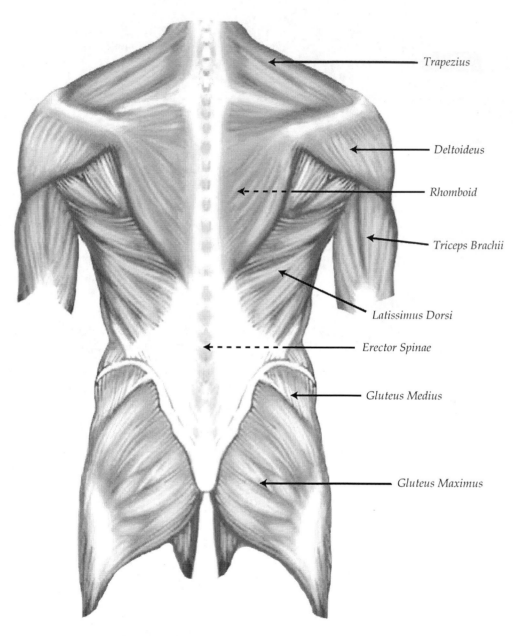

Trapezius

Deltoideus

Rhomboid

Triceps Brachii

Latissimus Dorsi

Erector Spinae

Gluteus Medius

Gluteus Maximus

Muscle Diagram 2. Posterior View (Back View)
[adapted from http://bsdweb.bsdvt.org/~aarchacki/pdfsMuscle%20Diagrams.pdf]

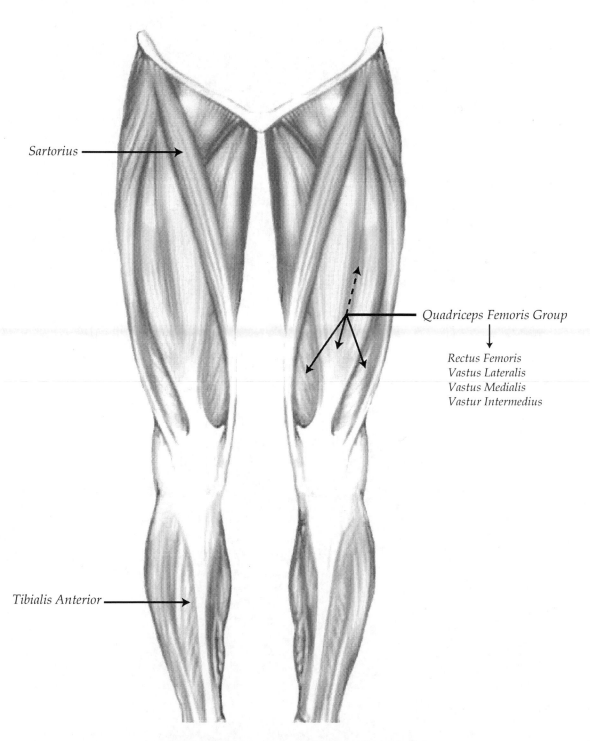

Sartorius

Quadriceps Femoris Group

Rectus Femoris
Vastus Lateralis
Vastus Medialis
Vastur Intermedius

Tibialis Anterior

Muscle Diagram 3. Anterior View (Front View)
[adapted from http://bsdweb.bsdvt.org/~aarchacki/pdfs/Muscle%20Diagrams.pdf]

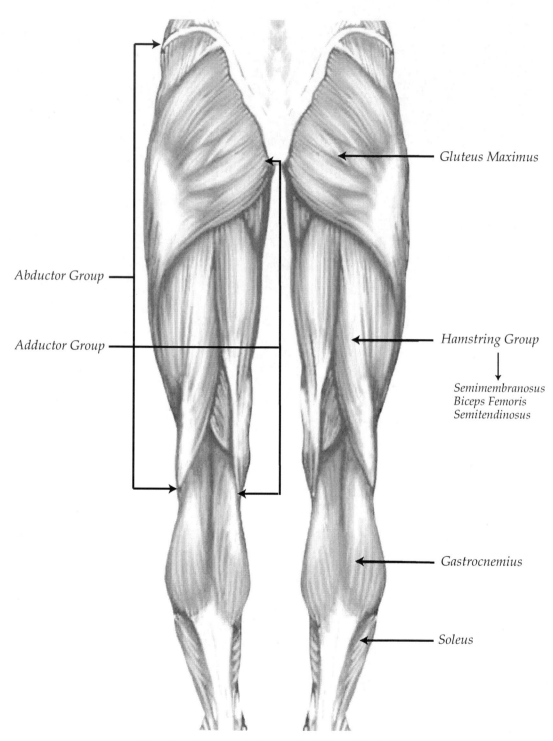

Gluteus Maximus

Abductor Group

Adductor Group

Hamstring Group

Semimembranosus
Biceps Femoris
Semitendinosus

Gastrocnemius

Soleus

Muscle Diagram 4. Posterior View (Back View)
[adapted from http://bsdweb.bsdvt.org/~aarchacki/pdfs/Muscle%20Diagrams.pdf]

Appendix G
MAT PILATES STUDY QUESTIONS I

TRUE/FALSE

_____ 1. Joseph Pilates immigrated to the United States from England.

_____ 2. Pilates stresses quality more than quantity.

_____ 3. Pilates may help prevent injuries because it helps to maintain a strong healthy body.

_____ 4. Pilates exercises can be done just about anywhere.

_____ 5. Breathing plays a major role in Pilates exercises.

_____ 6. The length and intensity of the warm up should be proportional to the intensity of the workout.

_____ 7. The advanced 100 should not be performed until the core muscles are conditioned to maintain proper body alignment.

_____ 8. Aerobic means without oxygen.

_____ 9. Abduction means to move away from the midline of the body.

_____ 10. Proper alignment is where bones and joints are symmetrically in line to avoid strain or injury.

FILL IN THE BLANK

_____ 11. _____ is lengthening or straightening

_____ 12. The mat work that Joseph Pilates developed while in one of the military camps was called _____.

_____ 13. Proper breathing in Pilates in breathing in through
                               the _____ and out through the _____.

_____ 14.

_____ 15. The "core" muscles consist of _____ and _____
                               muscles.

_____ 16.

_____ 17. All movements should be _____ and _____.

_____ 18.

_____ 19. _____ should be done when the muscles are
                               warm.

_____ 20. _____ stretching is the recommended method.

_____ 21. The _____ is a concept of introducing the Pilates
                               method and it's easy-to-learn exercises to people
                               with the hopes that they will individualize a prog-
                               ram to suit their needs.

_____ 22. The six essential nutrients are

_____ 23.

_____ 24.

_____ 25.

_____ 26.

_____ 27.

SHORT ANSWER

List and define the five components of fitness.

28. _____

_____

29. _____

_____

30. _____

_____

31. _____

_____

32. _____

_____

DEFINE

33. Frequency _____

34. Intensity _____

35. Time _____

MAT PILATES STUDY QUESTIONS II

Answer the following questions on a separate sheet of paper. Your answers should be typed and in complete sentences.

1. Explain the difference between aerobic and anaerobic exercises AND give two examples of each.

2. List the six essential nutrients that our body needs for survival AND a source of each.

3. Describe the process of beginning an exercise program (what safety issues must be addressed).

4. Describe the health benefits from participating in a regular exercise program. (Both physical and physiological effects)

5. Explain the acronym FITT and what it stands for.

6. Explain the concept of the basic equation CALORIES IN = CALORIES OUT formula and how to manipulate it for weight loss or gain.

7. Explain the term body composition and what does it tell us when it is tested.

8. Explain the difference between "pain" and "discomfort" in regards to exercising.

9. Explain the difference between muscular strength and muscular endurance.

10. Discuss the eating trends of Americans today AND how they have changed from the past?

11. Explain the term Basil Metabolic Rate.

12. List 3 exercises and the muscles being targeted.

13. Explain the difference between interval exercising (like body sculpting) and succession exercising.

14. Explain the concept of a circuit workout AND how it is set up?

15. List the items that must be included on a nutrition food label and why.

16. Explain the difference between Max Heart Rate and Target Heart Rate.

17. What information does our Target Heart Rate tell us when exercising AND how do we determine it?

18 Explain the purpose of a warm-up and cool-down AND how long should they be?

19. Explain the function of carbohydrates and why we need them in our diet.

20. Explain the two types of stretching and which is the preferred way to perform.

SECTION VII

REFERENCES

BOOKS/JOURNALS

Agatston, A. (2003). *South Beach Diet.* New York: Random House.

American Council on Exercise. (1996). *Lifestyle & Weight Management Consultant Manual 1st ed.* San Diego: American Council on Exercise.

Baechle, T. & Earle, R. (2005). *Weight Training: Steps to Success 3rd ed.* Champaign: Human Kinetics Publishing.

Bowden, B. & Bowden, J. 2002). *Illustrated Atlas of the Skeletal Muscles* .Englewood: Morton Publishing.

Boyle, M. & Zyla, G. (1992). *Personal Nutrition.* St. Paul: West Publishing Company.

Brown, S. P., Miller, W. C. & Eason, J. M. (2006). *Exercise Physiology basis of human movement in health and disease.* Baltimore: Lippincott Williams and Wilkins.

Colbert, D. (2007). *The Seven Pillars of Health.* Lake Mary, FA.: Siloam.

Craig, C. (2003). *Pilates on the Ball.* Rochester, Vermont: Healing Arts Press.

Cruise, J. (2005). *The 3 Hour Diet.* New York: Harper Collins Publishers.

Dillman, E. (2001). *The Little Book of Pilates.* New York: Warner books.

Earle, R. & Baechle, T. (2004). *NSCAS's Essentials of Personal Training.* Champaign: Human Kinetics.

Fahey, T. (2004). *Basic Weight Training for Men and Women 4th ed.* New York: McGraw Hill Publishing.

Gavin, J. (2002). *The Book of Pilates.* UAE: Paragon Publishing.

Hales, D. (2004). *An Invitation to Health.* Belmont: Thomson Wadsworth.

Kelly, E. (2001). *Common Sense Pilates.* London: Anness Publishing Limited.

Kravitz, L. (2006). *Anybody's Guide to Total Fitness 7th ed.* Dubuque: Kendall Hunt Publishing.

McArdle, W., Katch, F. & Katch, V. (2005). *Sports & Exercise Nutrition 2nd ed.* Baltimore: Lippincott Williams & Wilkins.

Menezes, A. (2000). *The Complete Guide to Joseph H. Pilates' Techniques of Physical Conditioning.* Alameda, CA: Hunter House Inc.

Pilates, J.H. & Miller, W.J. (1998). *Pilates' Return to Life Through Contrology.* Presentation Dynamics Inc.

Pilates, J.H. & Miller, W. J. (1934). *Your Health.* Presentation Dynamics Inc.

Powers, S., Dodd, S. & Noland, V. (2006). *Total Fitness and Wellness 4th ed.* San Francisco: Pearson Benjamin Cummings.

Roberts, H. *The Aspartame Problem. Statement for Commitment on Labor and Human Resources, U.S. Senate Hearing on "NutraSweet"- Health and Safety Concerns.* November 3, 1987. 83-178, U.S. Government Printing Office, Washington, 1988:466-467.

Siler, B. (2000). *The Pilates Body.* New York: Broadway Books.

Stewart, K. (2001). *Pilates for Beginners.* London: Carroll & Brown Publishing.

Ungaro, A. (2002). *Pilates Body in Motion.* New York: Dorling Kindersley.

Windsor, M. (1999). *The Pilates Power House.* New York: Perseus Books.

Wuest, D.A., & Bucher, C.A. (2006). *Foundations of Physical Education, Exercise Science, and Sport.* New York: McGraw-Hill.

ELECTRONIC SOURCES

A Body of Work, *Joseph H. Pilates,* 2006, www.abodyofwork-sf.com/josephh.pilates.html. Retrieved April 22, 2008.

All about Pilates, 2006, www.allaboutpilates.com/josephhubertus.htm. Retrieved April 22, 2008.

Cholesterol Management Health Center, 2007, http://www.webmd.com/ cholesterol-management/tc/High-Triglycerides-Overview. Retrieved April 22, 2008.

Crane, N., Hubbard, V. & Lewis, C. *American Diet sand Year 2000 Goals.* (1999) Retrieved February 26, 2007 from www.ers.usda.gov/publications/aib750/ aib750int.pdf.

Endurance Marketing Group. *15 Simple Ways to Improve Your Athletic Performance Now,* 2006, www.jdssportcoaching.com/15Ways.html.

Guthrie, J., Derby, B. & Levy, A. *What People Know and Do Not Know About Nutrition.* (1999) Retrieved February 26, 2007 from www.ers.usda.gov/publications/ aib750/aib750int.pdf.

Hale, J. (2005, December 1). Real strength training for boxers. Retrieved February 8, 2007 from http://www.bodybuilding.com/fun/hale7.htm.

Kennedy, E., Blaylock, J. & Kuhn, B. *On the Road to Better Nutrition.* (1999) Retrieved February 26, 2007 from www.ers.usda.gov/publications/aib750/aib750int.pdf.

Leduc, M. (2002). Triglycerides and the risk of stroke. http://www.healingdaily. com/conditions/triglycerides.htm. Retrieved April 22, 2008.

MayoClinic.com. (2005, March 4). Adjust your workout: Why warming up and cooling down keep you on the go. Retrieved February 5, 2007, from http:// www.cnn.com

Medismart, *Pilates,* 2006, www.medismart.com/pilates.htm.

Spring Training, *Pilates History,* 2006, www.spring-training.com/html/pilates history.html. Retrieved April 25, 2008.

Stern, J. *Dietary Trends.* Retrieved February 26, 2007 from www.ucdmc.ucdavis. edu/pulse/scripts/01_02/dietary_trends.pdf.

The Pilates Center, Method History, 2006, www.thepilatescenter.com/about/ methodhistory.cfm. Retrieved April 25, 2008.

Tippett, K. & Cleveland, L. *How Current Diets Stack Up.* (1999) Retrieved February 26, 2007 from www.ers.usda.gov/publications/aib750/aib750int.pdf.